Echocardiography
A Practical Guide for Reporting

Echocardiography
A Practical Guide for Reporting

Helen Rimington, BSc

Echocardiography Technician
Guy's & St Thomas' Hospitals, London, UK

John Chambers, MD, FRCP, FESC, FACC

Senior Lecturer and Consultant in Cardiology
Guy's & St Thomas' Hospitals, London, UK

The Parthenon Publishing Group
International Publishers in Medicine, Science & Technology

NEW YORK   LONDON

Library of Congress Cataloging-in-Publication Data

Rimington, Helen.
    Echocardiography : a practical guide for reporting / Helen Rimington and John Chambers.
        p.   cm.
    Includes bibliographical references and index.
    ISBN 1-85070-011-7
    1. Echocardiography—handbooks, manuals, etc.   I. Chambers, John, MD.   II. Title.
    [DNLM: 1. Echocardiography—handbooks.   2. Echocardiography—atlases.   3. Image Interpretation, Computer-Assisted—handbooks. WG 39 R576e 1997]
RC683.5.U5R55 1997
616.1'207543—dc21
DNLM/DLC   97-35746
for Library of Congress   CIP

British Library Cataloguing in Publication Data

    Rimington, Helen
    Echocardiography : a practical guide for reporting
    1. Echocardiography
    I. Title   II. Chambers, John, 1954–
    616.1'2'07543
    ISBN 1-85070-0117

Copyright © 1998
The Parthenon Publishing Group Limited

First published 1998

Published in North America by
The Parthenon Publishing Group Inc.
One Blue Hill Plaza
Pearl River
New York 10965, USA

Published in the UK and Europe by
The Parthenon Publishing Group Limited
Casterton Hall, Carnforth
Lancs. LA6 2LA, UK

Typeset by AMA Graphics Ltd., Preston, Lancashire, UK
Printed and bound in Spain by
T.G. Hostench, S. A.

Contents

Preface

There are many good comprehensive systematic textbooks of trans-thoracic echocardiography, but it may often be difficult to translate these into clinical practice. This guide will help the echocardiographer to write a clinically relevant report. It gives step-by-step advice about what to look for and how to interpret abnormal findings. Tables, line diagrams and Doppler recordings are used to clarify the text and a checklist for reporting is given in each chapter. This book will appeal to any technician or cardiologist studying for echocardiography certificates. It will also be useful as an aide-mémoire for established echocardiographers.

The left ventricle

LEFT VENTRICULAR SYSTOLIC FUNCTION

1. Regional wall motion

Look at each arterial region in every view (Figure 1.1). There are three components of motion: inward motion of the endocardium, wall thickening and phase. Inward motion can be affected by movement of adjacent territories and by swinging of the heart and respiratory motion. It is a good initial guide to abnormality, but systolic wall thickening is more reliable. These three components are summarized as wall motion (Table 1.1).

Table 1.1   Abnormalities of wall motion

Hypokinesis (< 50% normal movement)
Akinesis (absent movement)
Dyskinesis (movement out of phase with the rest of the ventricle)
Paradoxical (movement 180° out of phase)

2. Fractional shortening

This describes systolic function at the base of the heart. In the absence of regional wall motion abnormalities, this may reflect the rest of the left ventricle. It is usually calculated automatically from online software using M-mode left ventricular dimensions in diastole (LVDD) and systole (LVSD):

$$\text{Fractional shortening (\%)} = 100 \times (\text{LVDD} - \text{LVSD})/\text{LVDD}$$

3. Global function

Some measure of global function should be given. Any or all of the following may be used depending on the individual preference of your laboratory.

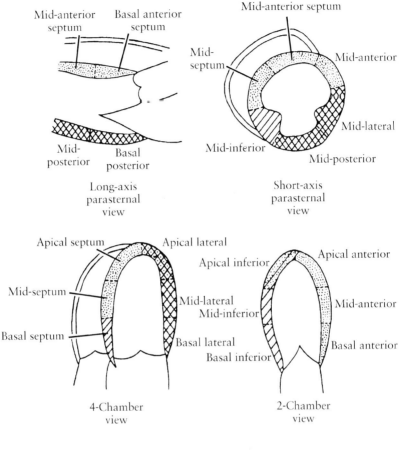

Left anterior descending distribution
Right coronary artery distribution
Circumflex distribution
Left anterior descending/circumflex overlap
Left anterior descending/right coronary artery overlap

Figure 1.1: Arterial territories of the heart: the motion of the endocardium within each arterial territory should be described (Table 1.1). Redrawn from Segar DS, *et al*. Dobutamine stress echocardiography: correlation with coronary lesion severity as determined by quantitative angiography. JACC 1992; 19:1197–1202 with permission of the Author and the Editors of the *Journal of the American College of Cardiology*

Ejection fraction

This can be estimated approximately as twice fractional shortening if there are no regional wall motion abnormalities. Otherwise, systolic and diastolic volumes should be calculated ideally using the biplane modified Simpson's rule (4- and 2-chamber views). Ejection fraction is then:

$$100 \times (\text{diastolic volume} - \text{systolic volume})/\text{diastolic volume}$$

With experience, ejection fraction can be estimated by eye. Whatever method is used, a value to the nearest 10% or a range (e.g. 40–50%) should be given, since the estimate can never be precise.

Systolic volume

Systolic volume is technically easier and more accurate to measure than diastolic volume. It provides prognostic information complementary to that obtained from ejection fraction. Normal ranges are given in Table 1.2[1-3].

Table 1.2 Normal adult ranges for left ventricular systolic function, 95% confidence interval (CI)

Fractional shortening (%)	28–44
Septal thickening (%)	18–53
Posterior wall thickening (%)	39–82
Ejection fraction (%)	60–80*
Stroke distance (cm)	15–35, 10–25 (elderly)
End-diastolic volume (ml)	< 166 (male), < 129 (female)
End-systolic volume (ml)	< 67 (male), < 59 (female)
4-chamber area diastole (cm²)	18.6–48.6
4-chamber area systole (cm²)	8.6–30.4

*In view of the inaccuracy inherent in making this estimation, an ejection fraction as low as 50% may be normal in some individuals

Stroke distance

Stroke distance is the same as the systolic velocity time integral (vti) and is measured using pulsed Doppler in the left ventricular outflow tract.

Stroke volume can be calculated from stroke distance using the left ventricular outflow tract diameter (d):

$$(\pi d^2/4) \times \text{vti}$$

Cardiac output is stroke volume × heart rate.

LEFT VENTRICULAR DIASTOLIC FUNCTION

1. Appearance on two dimensional imaging

Is there left ventricular hypertrophy or a large left atrium (in the absence of mitral valve disease), either of which suggests that diastolic function may be abnormal?

Is there abnormal density of the septum (suggesting amyloid or hypertrophic cardiomyopathy)?

2. Pattern of mitral filling

Place the pulsed sample at the level of the tips of the mitral leaflets in their fully open diastolic position. Measure the E deceleration time. Is the pattern of filling normal, slow or fast (restrictive)? (Figure 1.2). Normal ranges are given in Table 1.3[4-8].

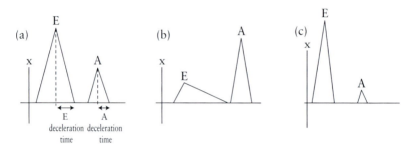

Figure 1.2:   Left ventricular filling patterns: (a) normal; (b) slow filling which means low peak E velocity, long deceleration time (and isovolumic relaxation period), high peak A velocity; (c) fast filling ('restrictive') which means high peak E velocity with short E deceleration time (and isovolumic relaxation time) and low or absent A wave. Isovolumic relaxation time is measured from the closing artifact of the aortic valve (x) to the start of transmitral flow

Table 1.3   Normal ranges for measures of diastolic function, 95% confidence interval (CI)

Mitral valve E (m/s)	0.4–1.0, 0.3–0.9 (elderly)
Mitral valve A (m/s)	0.2–0.6, 0.3–0.9 (elderly)
E : A ratio	0.7–3.1, 0.5–1.7 (elderly)
Mitral E deceleration time (ms)	139–219, 138–282 (elderly)
Mitral A deceleration time (ms)	> 70
IVRT (ms)	54–98, 56–124 (elderly)

IVRT, isovolumic relaxation time

If there is a fast (restrictive) pattern with a normal cavity size in diastole, consider restrictive cardiomyopathy versus constrictive pericarditis (pages 10–12)

3. If transmitral flow looks normal

This could be either genuinely normal or 'pseudonormal' as a result of underlying slow filling being modified by a high filling pressure.

- Place the sample volume about 1 cm into the right pulmonary vein in the apical 4-chamber view (Figure 1.3). Measure the peak velocity of pulmonary flow reversal and the relative heights of the systolic and diastolic filling waves (Figure 1.4) (Table 1.4)[4–9].

- Measure the transmitral A wave deceleration time (Table 1.4).

- Ask the patient to perform a Valsalva maneuver (hold the breath and bear down). As this is released, a slow filling pattern may be revealed in the presence of a pseudonormal transmitral flow pattern.

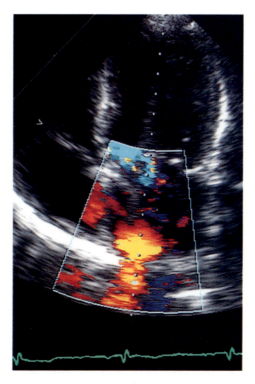

Figure 1.3: Recording pulmonary vein flow. The sample volume is placed 1 cm into the vein

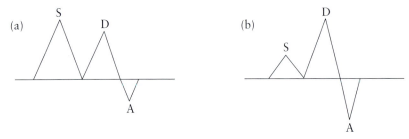

Figure 1.4: Pulmonary vein flow patterns: (a) normal; (b) high left ventricular diastolic pressure. S, systole; D, diastole; A, atrial flow reversal

Table 1.4 Doppler signs suggesting abnormal left ventricular diastolic function[9]

Mitral E wave deceleration time < 140 ms or > 280 ms
Mitral A wave deceleration time < 70 ms
E : A ratio < 0.7
Pulmonary vein systolic flow velocity < diastolic velocity
Pulmonary peak velocity during flow reversal > 0.35 m/s

THE LEFT VENTRICLE – PATTERNS IN CARDIOMYOPATHY

Secondary myocardial impairment (e.g. as a result of hypertension) cannot reliably be differentiated from the primary cardiomyopathies using echocardiography.

DILATED LEFT VENTRICLE

Table 1.5   Causes of dilated hypokinetic left ventricle

Myocardial infarction
Ischemic cardiomyopathy
Alcohol
Hypertension
End-stage aortic or mitral valve disease
Myocarditis
Dilated cardiomyopathy
Other e.g. Chagas' disease, sarcoid, hemachromatosis

---

1.   Diagnosis using cavity dimensions and systolic function

Visual appearance may be misleading and should be supplemented by cavity diameters on M-mode or 2D (pages 70–72).

Many conventional normal ranges are too low and may result in over-diagnosis of left ventricular dilatation especially in large subjects. Diastolic diameters as large as 5.9 cm may be normal (page 71).

Is the left ventricle hypokinetic (Table 1.5), normal or hyperkinetic? Borderline hypokinesis may occur in athletic hearts. If the left ventricle is hyperkinetic or in the upper normal range think of shunts or valve regurgitation (Table 1.6).

Table 1.6   Causes of left ventricular dilatation and hyperkinesis

---

Valve lesions
Aortic regurgitation
Mitral regurgitation

Shunts
Persistent ductus arteriosus
Aortopulmonary window
Sinus of Valsalva aneurysm
Ventricular septal defect

---

2. General appearance

Is there a regional abnormality suggesting an ischemic etiology?
Is there hypertrophy suggesting a hypertensive etiology or, less likely, hypertrophic cardiomyopathy?
Is the aortic or mitral valve abnormal in appearance or does the color flow Doppler map show regurgitation?

3. Filling patterns on pulsed Doppler

A fast (restrictive) pattern suggests a pulmonary artery wedge pressure > 20 mmHg and is associated with a poor prognosis.

4. Are there complications?

Look for:

- Thrombus.

- Functional mitral regurgitation.

- Pericardial fluid.

HYPERTROPHIED VENTRICLE (Table 1.7)

Table 1.7   Causes of hypertrophied left ventricle

Hypertension
Aortic stenosis
Hypertrophic cardiomyopathy (Table 1.8)
Amyloid (Table 1.9)
Athletic heart (Table 1.10)

Table 1.8   Features of hypertrophic cardiomyopathy

Left ventricular hypertrophy most frequently affecting the septum
Usually normal or hyperdynamic left ventricle (except end-stage)
Systolic anterior motion of anterior mitral leaflet
Intracavitary flow acceleration
Premature closure of aortic valve
Myocardial speckling

1. Diagnosis

The diagnosis of left ventricular hypertrophy in a patient with hypertension is usually made from wall thickness (page 70) supplemented by estimation of mass using M-mode dimensions (page 80) if there is no

Table 1.9   Features of amyloid

Myocardial hypertrophy (often including the right ventricle)
Sparkling myocardial appearance
Reduced cavity size
Reduced systolic function
Diffuse valve thickening
Biatrial enlargement

Table 1.10   Features of athletic heart

Mild left ventricular hypertrophy, septum usually around 1.3 cm
Mild left ventricular dilatation
Normal systolic function or mild global hypokinesis
Normal diastolic function

regional wall motion abnormality. Two-dimensional algorithms are more accurate but less frequently applied (pages 80 and 81).

In hypertrophic cardiomyopathy, the hypertrophy may be localized, thus invalidating generalized M-mode formulae for mass. Wall thickness should be measured at the base of the heart, but also at mid-cavity level and towards the apex or any other region that looks abnormal.

2. Geometry

- Concentric hypertrophy is defined as global hypertrophy with a small cavity size. It usually develops in response to pressure overload.

- Eccentric hypertrophy develops in response to left ventricular dilatation, for example as a result of severe aortic regurgitation. Wall thickness may be minimally increased, but because of the large cavity size, myocardial mass may be significantly increased (*see* formula on page 80).

3. Distribution

- Generalized hypertrophy affecting both right and left ventricles suggests amyloid or hypertrophic cardiomyopathy.

- Generalized left ventricular hypertrophy suggests hypertension.

- Localized hypertrophy, most commonly of the septum alone, suggests hypertrophic cardiomyopathy.

4. Severity of hypertrophy

- Minor hypertrophy may be found in restrictive myopathy (*see* below) or an athletic heart (septal width < 1.6 cm).

- Severe hypertrophy (septal width > 2 cm) usually suggests hypertrophic cardiomyopathy or amyloid, but may occasionally occur in hypertension (especially in West Indian subjects).

5. Is the myocardium echogenic?

Dense echogenicity suggests amyloid. Scattered echogenic spots are seen in hypertrophic cardiomyopathy but to some degree occur in hypertrophy from any cause.

6. Systolic function

Impaired systolic function with significant hypertrophy suggests amyloid rather than hypertrophic cardiomyopathy.

7. Filling patterns on pulsed Doppler

An abnormal slow filling pattern helps to differentiate pathological hypertrophy from athletic heart in which filling is normal.

A slow filling pattern may develop before significant left ventricular hypertrophy in hypertension.

8. Is there intracavitary or outflow tract flow acceleration?

This is assessed using continuous-wave Doppler from the apex (Figure 1.5).

Associated signs are systolic anterior motion of the anterior mitral leaflet, mitral regurgitation and early closure of the aortic valve.

NO HYPERTROPHY AND NO DILATATION

In a patient suspected of heart failure with an apparently normal ventricle, think of restrictive myopathy and constrictive pericarditis which can be differentiated as follows (Table 1.11)[10–13]:

1. Assess left atrial size, left ventricular wall thickness and ejection fraction

- In constriction, the atria and ejection fraction are usually normal.

- In restrictive myopathy, there may be biatrial enlargement, reduced systolic function and mild left ventricular hypertrophy.

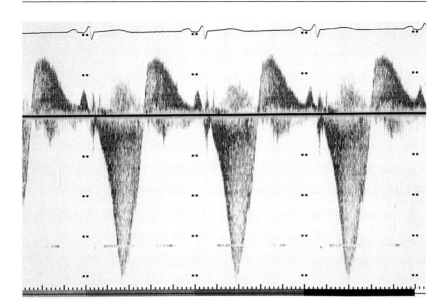

Figure 1.5: Dynamic flow acceleration in hypertrophic cardiomyopathy: this is caused by reduced cavity size and abnormal outflow tract geometry leading to high flow velocities developing in the latter part of systole

2. Measure respiratory variability of left-sided velocities

Use the transmitral E wave or continuous-wave aortic signal. Watch the chest to judge the respiratory cycle and measure the highest (expiratory) and lowest (inspiratory) peak velocities. There is a 10% difference in normal subjects, minor or absent variability in restriction and an exaggerated difference in constriction, usually > 40%.

3. Superior vena cava flow patterns

Diastolic abnormalities are shown by greater than average flow reversal (Figure 1.6).

Table 1.11   Differentiation of restrictive myopathy and pericardial constriction

	Restrictive myopathy	*Pericardial constriction*
Shared characteristics		
Transmitral flow	short deceleration time	
LV filling	early cessation	
SVC reverse flow	increased	
Differences		
Pericardium	normal	may be thickened
Left atrium	large	usually normal
LV ejection fraction	low	normal
Respiratory variability of left-sided flow	none	large (> 40%)
SVC forward flow	dominant in diastole	variable
SVC reverse flow	increased in inspiration	increased in expiration
PEP/EJT	> 0.5	< 0.4

LV, left ventricular; SVC, superior vena cava; PEP, measured from the Q wave to the aortic valve opening artifact; EJT, measured from aortic opening to closing artifact

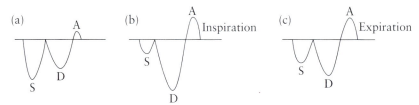

Figure 1.6:   Superior vena cava flow patterns: (a) normal. There is dominant systolic forward flow with minor reversal during atrial systole on expiration; (b) restrictive myopathy. There is dominant diastolic forward flow with increased reversal on inspiration; (c) pericardial constriction. Forward flow patterns vary from normal to systolic or diastolic dominance. The characteristic feature is increased flow reversal during atrial systole maximal in expiration. S, systole; D, diastole; A, atrial flow reversal

REPORTING LEFT VENTRICULAR FUNCTION

1. **Left ventricular dimensions**
2. **Systolic function – regional**
                          global
3. **Diastolic function**
4. **Specific features, e.g. systolic anterior motion of the mitral valve**
5. **Complications, e.g. thrombus, mitral regurgitation**
6. **Right ventricular function and pulmonary artery pressure**
7. **Any valve disease**

COMMON MISTAKES

Overdiagnosis of hypertrophic cardiomyopathy

A subaortic septal bulge is common in patients aged over 65 years. Artifactual hypertrophy may be produced by foreshortening the left ventricle in an off-axis view. Remember that there are other causes of left ventricular hypertrophy including hypertension.

There may be mild outflow acceleration in left ventricular hypertrophy of any cause.

Hypertrophic cardiomyopathy versus aortic stenosis

Left ventricular hypertrophy induced by aortic stenosis can cause dynamic outflow obstruction, especially if the patient is underfilled or the left ventricle is stimulated, for example, by dobutamine.

Conversely, hypertrophic cardiomyopathy can cause thickening of the aortic valve as a result of turbulence in the left ventricular outflow tract. This can become a focus for the development of endocarditis.

Athletic heart versus hypertrophic cardiomyopathy

The differential echocardiographic features are given in Tables 1.8 and 1.10. Athletic heart has a dilated cavity, symmetric hypertrophy and normal diastolic function. Hypertrophic cardiomyopathy typically has asymmetric hypertrophy, a small cavity and abnormal diastolic function. In addition, athletic heart is associated with a normal electrocardiogram while hypertrophic cardiomyopathy is associated with increased voltages and T-wave abnormalities. There is no family history in athletic heart, and the left ventricular hypertrophy regresses after cessation of training.

Echocardiogram apparently normal despite suspected heart failure

In the absence of abnormal left ventricular systolic function, check for diastolic left ventricular dysfunction, right ventricular function and pulmonary hypertension.

REFERENCES

1. Rawles J. In *Echocardiography: an International Review*. JB Chambers, M Monaghan (Eds). 1993. Oxford: Oxford University Press. pp 23–36
2. Pearlman JD, Triulzi MO, King ME, *et al*. Limits of normal left ventricular dimensions in growth and development; analysis of dimensions and variance in the two dimensional echocardiograms in 268 normal healthy subjects. *JACC* 1988; 12: 1432–41
3. Schiller NB, Foster E. Analysis of left ventricular systolic function. *Heart* 1996; 75 (Suppl 2). 17–26
4. Zarich SW, Arbuckle BE, Cohen LR, *et al*. Diastolic abnormalities in young asymptomatic diabetic patients assessed by pulsed Doppler echocardiography. *JACC* 1988; 12: 114–30
5. Van Dam I, Fast J, DeBono T. Normal diastolic filling patterns of the left ventricle. *Eur Heart J* 1988; 9: 165–71
6. Sagie A, Benjamin EJ, Galderisi M, *et al*. Reference values for Doppler indices of left ventricular diastolic filling in the elderly. *J Am Soc Echocard* 1993; 6: 570–6
7. Tenenbaum A, Motro A, Hod H, *et al*. Shortened Doppler-derived mitral A wave deceleration time; an important predictor of elevated left ventricular filling pressure. *JACC* 1996; 27: 700–5
8. Cohen GI, Pietrolungo JF, Thomas JD. A practical guide to assessment of ventricular diastolic function using Doppler echocardiography. *JACC* 1996; 27: 1753–60
9. Giannuzzi P, Temporelli PL, Bosimini E, *et al*. Independent and incremental prognostic value of Doppler-derived mitral deceleration time of early filling in both symptomatic and asymptomatic patients with left ventricular dysfunction. *JACC* 1996; 28: 383–90
10. Armstrong TG, Lewis BS, Gotsman MS. Systolic time intervals in constrictive pericarditis and primary myocardial disease. *Am Heart J* 1973; 85: 6–12
11. Khuller S, Lewis RP. Usefulness of systolic time intervals in differential diagnosis of constrictive pericarditis and restrictive myopathy. *Br Heart J* 1976; 38: 43–6
12. Ghose JC, Mitra SK, Chetri MK. Systolic time intervals in the differential diagnosis of constrictive pericarditis and cardiomyopathy. *Br Heart J* 1976; 38: 47–50
13. Appleton C, Hatle L, Popp R. Demonstration of restrictive ventricular physiology by Doppler echocardiography. *JACC* 1988; 11: 757–68

𝟤

Myocardial infarction

1. Regional systolic function

- The diagnosis is confirmed by a regional abnormality.

- Comment on the other regions. Compensatory hyperkinesis is a good prognostic sign. Hypokinesis of a territory other than of the acute infarct suggests multivessel disease and is a poor prognostic sign.

- If there is an inferior infarct check the right ventricle. About 10% of all inferior infarcts are associated with significant right ventricular infarction.

2. Global systolic function

This gives prognostic information. The ejection fraction is still traditionally used to guide the use of angiotensin-converting enzyme inhibitors (for example a threshold of < 40% is often applied).

3. Diastolic function (page 4)

4. Complications

Check for these (Table 2.1) in all cases.

Table 2.1 Complications after myocardial infarction

Thrombus (Table 2.2)
Aneurysm
Pseudoaneurysm
Mitral regurgitation
Ventricular septal rupture

- If there is a murmur check for mitral regurgitation and ventricular septal rupture. These may coexist. If there is mitral regurgitation, consider the causes in Table 2.3.

Table 2.2 Features of thrombus

Underlying wall motion abnormality
Cleavage plane between thrombus and left ventricular wall
Higher density than normal myocardium
Usually visible in more than one echocardiographic section

Table 2.3 Causes of mitral regurgitation after myocardial infarction

Rupture of chordae
Rupture of papillary muscle
Restricted mitral leaflet (Figure 2.1)
Left ventricular dilatation
Mitral prolapse
Coexistent mitral valve disease

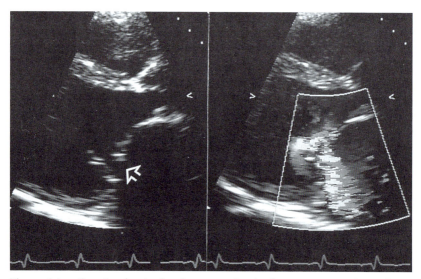

Figure 2.1: Restricted mitral valve: posterior leaflet restriction after inferior myocardial infarction is caused by failure of the base of the heart to shorten during systole. This in turn means that the mitral annulus can no longer move towards the apex and the posterior leaflet is prevented from falling back into the plane of the annulus (arrow; left-hand panel). The resulting jet of regurgitation is directed behind the posterior leaflet (right hand panel) (i.e. in the direction opposite to mitral prolapse)

- Complete or partial rupture of the papillary muscle or septal rupture should be reported directly to the clinician responsible for the case.

- A true aneurysm complicates about 5% of all anterior infarcts and is a sign of a poor prognosis. It must be distinguished from a false aneurysm caused by free wall rupture contained by the pericardium (Table 2.4) (Figure 2.2).

Table 2.4 Differentiation of true and pseudoaneurysm

	True aneurysm	*Pseudoaneurysm*
Position	usually apical	usually posterior
Neck	wide	narrow
Color flow	usually absent	into in systole, out of in diastole

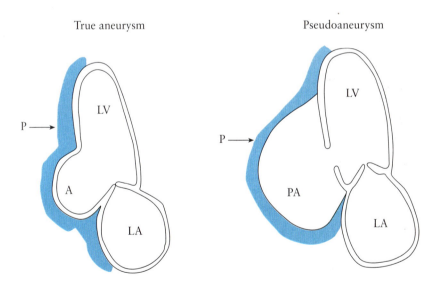

Figure 2.2: True and pseudoaneurysm: a true aneurysm (left) has a wide neck; a pseudoaneurysm (right) has a narrow neck through which blood enters in systole and leaves in diastole. A, aneurysm; PA, pseudoaneurysm; LA, left atrium; LV, left ventricle; P, pericardium

REPORTING MYOCARDIAL INFARCTION

1. Regional wall motion
2. Global systolic function
3. Diastolic function
4. Complications

3

Aortic valve disease

AORTIC STENOSIS

1. Appearance of valve

Look at the number of cusps, pattern of thickening and mobility. These may give a clue to the etiology (Table 3.1).

Table 3.1 Clues to etiology in aortic stenosis

	Systolic bowing	Closure line	Associated features
Calcific degeneration	no	central	—
Bicuspid	yes	eccentric	ascending aortic dilatation; coarctation
Rheumatic	yes	central	mitral involvement

2. Assess left ventricle

Look for left ventricular hypertrophy which suggests (but does not prove) severe stenosis. If the left ventricle is impaired, the transaortic pressure difference may underestimate the severity of the stenosis and you should apply the continuity equation.

3. Doppler measurements

- Measure the continuous waveform from the apex and at least one other approach (suprasternal or right intercostal).

- If the Vmax is < 3.0 m/s, use the long form of the Bernoulli equation (page 79). This will require a pulsed measurement in the left ventricular outflow tract in the 5-chamber view (Figure 3.1).

- Use the continuity equation (page 79) to calculate effective orifice area if:

    The peak transaortic velocity is 3.0–4.5 m/s (to help differentiate moderate from severe stenosis).

19

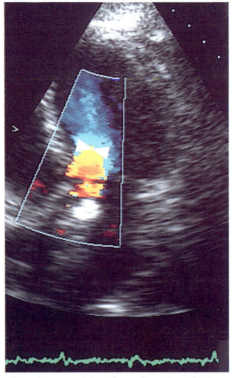

Figure 3.1: Sample volume position for subaortic velocity recording: this is a 5-chamber view. The pulsed sample is moved up and down in the left ventricular outflow tract until waveforms are found immediately before a sudden step-up in velocity or before aliasing begins

The peak transaortic velocity is < 3.0 m/s but the left ventricle is impaired.

• Assess severity (Table 3.2).

4. General

Assess:

• The degree of aortic regurgitation (page 25, Table 3.4).

• The other valves.

• Aortic root dilatation and coarctation if the aortic valve is bicuspid.

Table 3.2 Severity in aortic stenosis

	Mild	Moderate to severe*	Critical
Aortic Vmax (m/s)	2.0–3.0	3.0–4.5	>4.5
Peak gradient (mmHg)	<40	40–80	>80
Mean gradient (mmHg)	<20	20–50	>50
EOA (continuity equation) (cm²)	>1.0	0.6–1.0	<0.6

*Moderate and severe stenosis can be difficult to distinguish because of the influence of left ventricular function as well as individual patient's susceptibility. Classification in this range may need to take account of clinical findings. EOA, effective orifice area; Vmax, peak velocity

- Right ventricular function and pulmonary pressure. Pulmonary hypertension is a grave sign in severe aortic stenosis. It must be assessed if the aortic stenosis is severe or if the left or right ventricle is impaired.

REPORTING AORTIC STENOSIS

1. **Left ventricular dimensions and systolic function**
2. **Appearance of the aortic valve**
3. **Severity of stenosis**
4. **Other valves**
5. **Right ventricular function (pulmonary artery pressure if indicated)**

COMMON MISTAKES

Subaortic membrane (Figure 3.2)

This is suggested if there is evidence of a fixed stenosis on continuous-wave Doppler recordings, but the aortic valve is disproportionately mobile. Aortic valve thickening is caused by turbulence in the left ventricular outflow tract beyond the membrane.

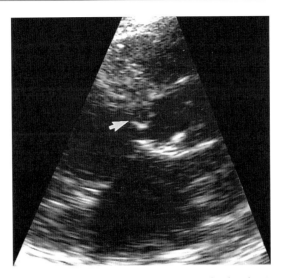

Figure 3.2: Subaortic membrane: this is easily missed. The clue is a discrepancy between high left ventricular outflow tract velocities and a mobile aortic valve

Poor left ventricle and aortic stenosis of uncertain severity

It may be difficult to differentiate critical aortic stenosis causing left ventricular impairment and less severe stenosis with a poor left ventricle as a result of another etiology. Either may cause a low transaortic pressure difference associated with a small effective orifice area. The problem may be resolved by advanced techniques including stress echocardiography.

AORTIC REGURGITATION

1. Appearance of valve and aortic root

This may allow you to determine the etiology (Table 3.3).

Table 3.3   Etiology in aortic regurgitation

Aortic root
    dilatation
    dissection
 	
 Valve
    bicuspid
    rheumatic
    calcific degeneration
    endocarditis
    prolapse
    diaphenous (normal echocardiographic thickness)
    others, e.g. SLE

SLE, systemic lupus erythematosus

2. Color flow mapping

The height of the jet measured about 0.5 cm below the cusps reflects the size of the regurgitant orifice. When expressed as a percentage of the height of the left ventricular outflow tract, it gives an empirical measure of the degree of regurgitation. For a central jet this measurement is most accurately made using color M-mode (Figure 3.3).

3. Continuous-wave signal

Record using a stand-alone probe either from the apex or, if the jet is directed posteriorly, from the parasternal position.

Look at the slope or pressure half-time (Figure 3.4) and the density of the signal compared with the density of forward flow.

4. The left ventricle

Answer these questions:

• Is there volume load (suggesting severe aortic regurgitation)? Chronic severe regurgitation usually causes a diastolic diameter > 6.0 cm.

• What is the fractional shortening? If < 25%, the outcome even after surgery is likely to be poor.

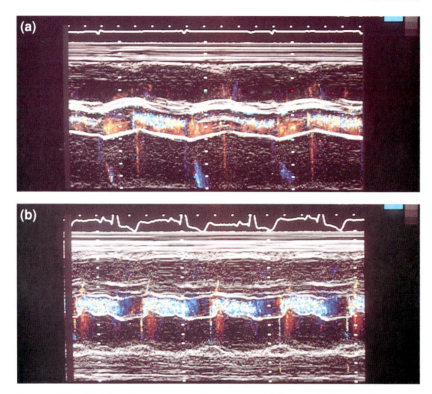

Figure 3.3: Height of aortic regurgitant jet and left ventricular outflow tract: the height of the color flow map is expressed as a percentage of the outflow tract height. In (a) the regurgitation is moderate; in (b) it is severe

5. Severity of regurgitation

- Use color and continuous-wave ultrasound (Table 3.4)[1-3]. Also, take into account the size and activity of the left ventricle.

- If there is doubt, image the aorta looking for diastolic flow reversal. Reversal in the arch suggests at least moderate regurgitation, reversal in the descending thoracic aorta suggests severe regurgitation (Figure 3.5).

6. General

Assess:

- The other valves.

- The right ventricle.

- The rest of the aorta if the ascending aorta is dilated.

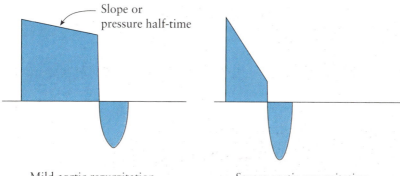

Slope or
pressure half-time

Mild aortic regurgitation   Severe aortic regurgitation

Figure 3.4: Measurement of the pressure half-time and slope of the aortic regurgitant jet continuous-wave Doppler signal: in severe aortic regurgitation, the end-diastolic left ventricular pressure and aortic pressure approximate so the driving pressure and, therefore, the end-diastolic velocity of the continuous-wave signal are low. The peak velocity remains approximately normal so that the slope of the waveform is steep. The pressure half-time may also be calculated by analogy with the diastolic signal in mitral stenosis. The signal in mild regurgitation is shown on the left and in severe regurgitation on the right

Table 3.4   Criteria of severity in aortic regurgitation

	Mild*	Moderate*	Severe
Continuous-wave slope (m/s^2)	< 2.0	1.5–3.0	> 3.0
Continuous-wave pressure half-time (ms)	> 500	400–600	< 400
Color/LVOT height (%)	< 25	25–60	> 60

*Mild and moderate regurgitation cannot reliably be differentiated. LVOT, left ventricular outflow tract

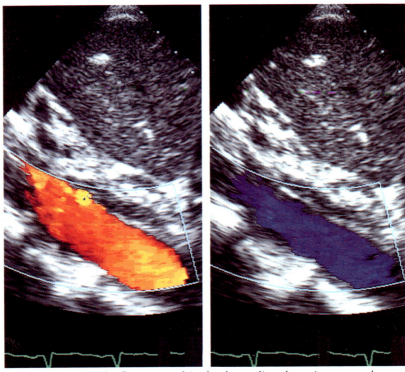

Figure 3.5: Diastolic flow reversal in the descending thoracic aorta or beyond suggests severe aortic regurgitation. In this case, the right-hand panel shows reversed flow in the abdominal aorta. Forward flow is shown in the left-hand panel

REPORTING AORTIC REGURGITATION

1. **Dimensions of left ventricle and aorta**
2. **Etiology**
3. **Severity**
4. **Left ventricular function**
5. **Other valves**

COMMON MISTAKES

Steep continuous-wave slope and narrow color jet

Steep slopes occur in severe regurgitation, but also in more mild regurgitation if the left ventricle is impaired with a high end-diastolic pressure from another cause (e.g. myocardial infarction) (Figure 3.6).

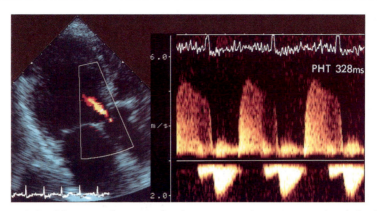

Figure 3.6: Narrow color map despite steep continuous-wave signal: in this patient with an inferior infarct, there is a thin jet of aortic regurgitation on color flow mapping (left-hand panel). The pressure half-time of the continuous-wave signal (right-hand panel) is 330 ms which is consistent with either severe regurgitation or, more likely in the clinical context, a high left ventricular diastolic pressure

REFERENCES

1. Perry GJ, Helmcke F, Nanda NC, *et al*. Evaluation of aortic insufficiency by color Doppler flow mapping. *JACC* 1987; 9: 952–9
2. Teague SM, Heinsimer JA, Anderson JL, *et al*. Quantification of aortic regurgitation utilizing continuous wave Doppler ultrasound. *JACC* 1986; 8: 592–9
3. Samstad SO, Hagrenaes L, Skjaerpe T, *et al*. Half-time of the diastolic aortoventricular pressure difference by continuous wave Doppler ultrasound: a measure of the severity of aortic regurgitation? *Br Heart J* 1989; 61: 336–42

4

Mitral valve disease

MITRAL STENOSIS

1. Appearance of valve

Assess:

- The distribution and degree of thickening of each leaflet.
- Whether there is calcification in the line of commissural fusion.
- The mobility of the anterior and posterior leaflets.
- The degree of chordal involvement.

2. Planimeter mitral valve orifice area (Figure 4.1)

- Make sure that the section is not oblique.
- Take care not to planimeter the chordae which, if thickened, can mimic the orifice.
- Use color flow Doppler as a guide to the extent of the orifice if this is not obvious on imaging. If there is significant reverberation artifact, the measurement may be inaccurate and should not be made.

3. Continuous-wave signal

Measure the pressure half-time and mean gradient, averaging at least five cycles if there is atrial fibrillation.

Estimate pulmonary artery pressure (pages 49–50).

4. Assess severity (Table 4.1)

5. Assess mitral regurgitation (pages 32–35)

Anything more than mild regurgitation precludes balloon valvotomy.

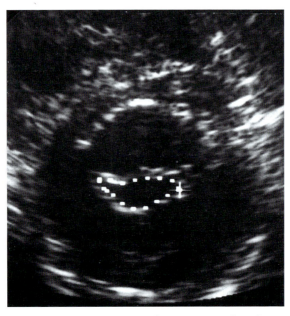

Figure 4.1: Planimetry of the mitral orifice: care must be taken to section the tips of the mitral leaflets perpendicularly. A common mistake is to section towards the base of the leaflets or across thickened chordae

Table 4.1   Criteria of severity in mitral stenosis

	Mild	*Moderate*	*Severe*
Planimetered OA (cm²)	> 1.5	1.0–1.5	< 1.0
Pressure half-time (ms)	< 150	150–200	> 200
Mean gradient (mmHg)	< 5	5–10	> 10
PA systolic pressure*(mmHg)	25	25–35	> 35

*PA systolic pressure has a variable relationship to severity of stenosis; OA, orifice area; PA, pulmonary artery

6. Assess other valves

Severe aortic regurgitation tends to shorten mitral pressure half-time.

7. Right ventricular function

A failing right ventricle is an indication for invasive intervention even if there is relatively minor breathlessness.

8. Is there intra-atrial thrombus?

Transthoracic echocardiography is insensitive for detecting thrombus. A transesophageal study should always be performed before balloon valvotomy.

9. Is the valve amenable to balloon valvotomy? (Table 4.2)[1,2]

A score of 1–4 can be given for each of valve tip calcification, thickening of the leaflet base, leaflet mobility and chordal involvement. A total score above 8 suggests a low success, but is not completely reliable. Commissural calcification is associated with a high rate of leaflet tearing.

Table 4.2 Criteria for valvotomy

Thickening largely confined to leaflet tips
Good mobility of anterior leaflet
Little chordal involvement
No more than mild mitral regurgitation
No left atrial thrombus ·
No commissural calcification

REPORTING MITRAL STENOSIS

1. **Appearance of valve**
2. **Severity**
3. **Right-sided pressures and right ventricular function**
4. **Is the valve amenable to balloon valvotomy?**
5. **Other valves**

COMMON MISTAKES

Mitral annular calcification versus mitral stenosis

It may be difficult to image the leaflets if there is dense reverberation artifact from mitral annular calcification. The leaflets are usually more easily seen in the apical views and there will be no evidence of obstruction on Doppler.

MITRAL REGURGITATION

1. Appearance and movement of valve

Answer the following questions to determine the etiology (Table 4.3):

- What is the distribution and degree of any leaflet thickening? Rheumatic thickening primarily involves the tips; in systemic lupus erythematosus, there is more generalized thickening.

- Is there a discrete echogenic mass (e.g. vegetation)?

- Does the valve open normally during diastole or is there bowing of the leaflets suggesting rheumatic disease?

- Is there evidence of leaflet prolapse? (Table 4.4)

- Are there redundant cuspal or chordal echoes (suggesting a floppy valve)?

- Is there restriction of motion of the posterior leaflet during systole? (Table 4.5)

Table 4.3   Etiology of mitral regurgitation

Ischemic
   restricted posterior leaflet
   prolapse
   papillary muscle rupture or dysfunction
Functional
Floppy mitral valve
Rheumatic
Endocarditis
Other, e.g. systemic lupus erythematosus

Table 4.4   Signs of prolapse (Figure 4.2)

Movement of any part of either leaflet behind the plane of the annulus in the long-axis view
Movement of the point of coaption behind the plane of the annulus in the 4-chamber view
Usually, the jet is directed away from the prolapsing leaflet

---

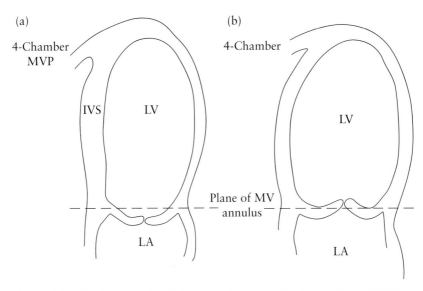

Figure 4.2: Prolapse: in the 4-chamber view, mitral valve prolapse (MVP) is diagnosed if there is movement of the point of apposition of the valve into the left atrium during systole (a). Buckling of the leaflets alone (b) is within normal limits. LA, left atrium; LV, left ventricle; IVS, interventricular septum

---

Table 4.5   Restriction of posterior leaflet motion (Figure 2.1)

Tip of leaflet held in the left ventricle during systole
Inferior infarct causing failure of shortening of left ventricle in
  systole
Jet directed posteriorly

---

2. Color flow Doppler mapping (Figure 4.3) (Table 4.6)

Assess:

- The size of the flow recruitment area in the left ventricle.

- The width of the base of the jet at the level of the valve.

- The intra-atrial jet area if the jet is central. The size of an eccentric jet will be modified by interactions with the left atrial wall.

- The location of the base of the jet (usually from the parasternal short-axis view).

- The direction of the jet (away from a prolapsing leaflet, behind a restricted leaflet).

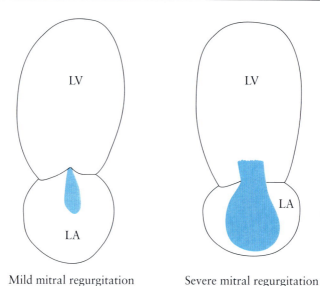

Mild mitral regurgitation   Severe mitral regurgitation

Figure 4.3: Diagram of a mitral regurgitant jet: a significant jet consists of a region of flow recruitment in the left ventricle, a neck level with the valve and an intra-atrial portion. The intra-atrial jet size is dependent on mechanical changes within the left atrium, for example loss of momentum caused by striking the left atrial wall. The flow recruitment area and neck may, therefore, give more reliable estimates of severity. The left-hand panel shows mild and the right-hand panel severe mitral regurgitation. LA, left atrium; LV, left ventricle

Table 4.6   Indicators of degree of mitral regurgitation[3]

	Mild ➝	*Severe*
Jet width at base (cm)	< 0.5	> 1
Jet area (cm²)	< 4.0	> 8.0
Flow recruitment	none	++
Density on continuous wave	+	++
Duration	can be short	holosystolic
Pulmonary vein systolic flow	normal blunted	reversed
Pulmonary artery pressure	normal	up to 50 mmHg

3. Continuous-wave Doppler

Look at the shape and density of the signal:

- A signal as dense as forward flow suggests severe regurgitation. Mild regurgitation is associated with an incomplete outline or a low-intensity signal.

- A rapid rise in left atrial pressure in severe regurgitation causes an early descent of the Doppler signal. In extreme cases, the signal may resemble a recording across the aortic valve.

4. Left ventricular function

Assess:

- The cavity dimensions and fractional shortening. Severe mitral regurgitation usually causes a high fractional shortening, but as myocardial fibrosis and failure supervene, the fractional shortening falls. A value below 29% suggests that recovery after surgery is unlikely.

- Regional function. Restriction of the posterior leaflet is a complication of an inferior infarct.

5. Other guides to severity

- An elevated pulmonary artery pressure which may be as high as about 50 mmHg in severe regurgitation.

- Abnormal systolic pulmonary vein flow (blunting in moderate regurgitation, reversal in severe regurgitation).

REPORTING MITRAL REGURGITATION

1. **Etiology of mitral regurgitation**
2. **Severity**
3. **Left ventricular dimensions and systolic function**
4. **Pulmonary artery pressure**
5. **Other valve disease?**
6. **Is the valve repairable?**

COMMON MISTAKES

Eccentric jet

If the jet hugs the wall of the left atrium, it will stretch out and become thinned in one plane and broadened in the orthogonal plane. Its area is then a particularly poor guide to severity. However, the intraventricular flow recruitment area and the base of the jet remain reliable as do the indirect signs including the pattern of pulmonary vein flow.

Overdiagnosis of mitral prolapse

Buckling of the leaflets is normal on the apical 4-chamber view, but may mistakenly be diagnosed as prolapse (*see* Table 4.4 and Figure 4.2).

REFERENCES

1. Wilkins GT, Weyman AE, Abascal VM, *et al*. Percutaneous balloon dilatation of the mitral valve: an analysis of echocardiographic variables related to outcome and the mechanism of dilatation. *Br Heart J* 1988; 60: 299–308
2. Cannan CR, Nishimura RA, Reeder GS, *et al*. Echocardiographic assessment of commissural calcium: a simple predictor of outcome after percutaneous mitral balloon valvotomy. *JACC* 1997; 29: 175–80
3. Spain MG, Grayburn PA, Harlamert EA, *et al*. Quantitive assessment of mitral regurgitation by Doppler color flow imaging: angiographic and hemodynamic correlations. *JACC* 1989; 13: 585–90

5

Prosthetic valves

1. Appearance of valve
- Position and type (Figures 5.1 and 5.2) (Table 5.1);
- Does the prosthesis rock? In the aortic position this is always caused by dehiscence. In the mitral position rocking may be normal.

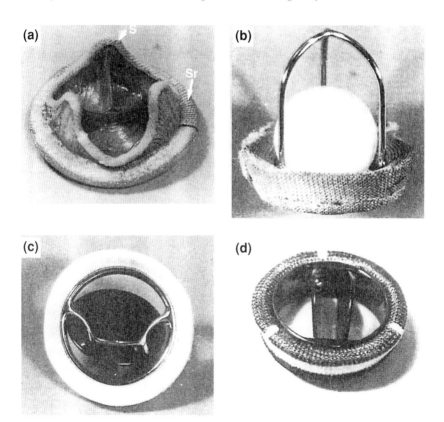

Figure 5.1: Photographs of prosthetic valve types: (a) porcine; (b) caged ball; (c) tilting disc; (d) bileaflet. sr, sewing ring; s, stent

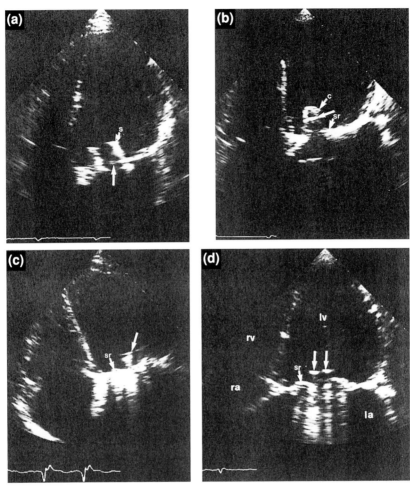

Figure 5.2: Echo images of prosthetic valve types: 4-chamber views illustrating (a) a porcine xenograft (cusp arrowed); (b) a caged ball valve (ball arrowed); (c) a tilting disc valve (disc arrowed); and (d) a bileaflet prosthesis (both leaflets arrowed). sr, sewing ring; s, strut; c, cage; la, left atrium; lv, left ventricle; ra, right atrium; rv, right ventricle

If valve is biological

- Are the cusps thickened (> 3 mm in thickness)?

- Is there a separate echogenic mass (either vegetation or torn cusp)?

- Is cusp motion normal or is there decreased motion (suggesting obstruction) or increased motion (suggesting a tear)? A small tear will cause prolapse; a larger tear will result in a flail cusp or segment.

Table 5.1 Types of replacement heart valve

Biological
Autograft
Homograft
Xenograft
   stented (Figure 5.2a)
      porcine e.g. Hancock, Carpentier–Edwards
      pericardial usually bovine, e.g. Baxter
   stentless, e.g. St Jude Toronto, Baxter Prima

Mechanical
   caged ball (Figure 5.2b), e.g. Starr–Edwards
   tilting disc (Figure 5.2c), e.g. Bjork Shiley, Medtronic Hall
   bileaflet (Figure 5.2d), e.g. St Jude Medical, Carbomedics, ATS,
      Sorin bicarbon

If valve is mechanical

- Does the occluder open quickly and to its full extent?

- If there are two leaflets, do both open equally?

2. Is there any regurgitation?

Replacement valve in aortic position

- How many jets are there?

- Is the regurgitation through the valve or paraprosthetic?

Mild leakage through a mechanical prosthesis is normal. In bileaflet valves, there can be up to four jets with their origin at the pivots near the edge of the orifice. Tilting disc valves have two regurgitant jets. A normal Starr–Edwards valve has a trivial central jet.

The base of a paraprosthetic jet is outside the sewing ring. Its site can be described by analogy with a clock face using the parasternal short-axis view.

Replacement valve in mitral position

- An easily-seen jet is usually paraprosthetic since normal trans-prosthetic regurgitation tends to be hidden by flow shielding.

- The intraventricular flow recruitment region of paraprosthetic regurgitation can usually be seen even when the intra-atrial jet is invisible.

- If valve dysfunction is suspected and the transthoracic study is normal, transesophageal echocardiography must be performed.

3. Severity of regurgitation

- Use the same methods as for native regurgitation (pages 23–27, 32–35). For valves in the aortic position, assessing the height of a jet relative to the left ventricular outflow tract diameter may be difficult since paraprosthetic jets are often eccentric.

- The circumference of the sewing ring occupied by the jet is another guide for valves in both the aortic and mitral positions: mild (< 10%), moderate (10–25%), severe (> 25%).

- Transesophageal echocardiography is usually necessary to assess severity of regurgitation for mechanical valves in the mitral position.

4. Forward flow

Measurements needed are given in Table 5.2.

- Normal ranges vary by valve type, size and position (pages 74–78).

- The pressure half-time orifice area method is not valid for normally functioning valves in the mitral position.

Table 5.2   Measurements necessary to assess forward flow

Aortic position	peak velocity
	calculated mean and peak gradient
	effective orifice area by classical form of continuity equation (page 79)
Mitral position	peak velocity
	mean gradient
	pressure half-time

5. Are there signs of obstruction?

Signs suggesting obstruction are given in Table 5.3[1].

- Reduced cusp or occluder motion are the most reliable signs, particularly for valves in the mitral position.

- High derived gradients are common in normally functioning 19 mm or 21 mm prostheses in the aortic position.

- Progressive changes or a change from immediate postoperative values are more valuable than a single result.

Table 5.3 Signs suggesting obstruction

Aortic	EOA < 1.0 cm^2 in valve > 21 mm in diameter fall in effective orifice area of 30% since postoperative study
Mitral	pressure half-time > 200 ms with peak velocity > 2.5 m/s
Tricuspid	peak velocity > 1.5 m/s

EOA, effective orifice area

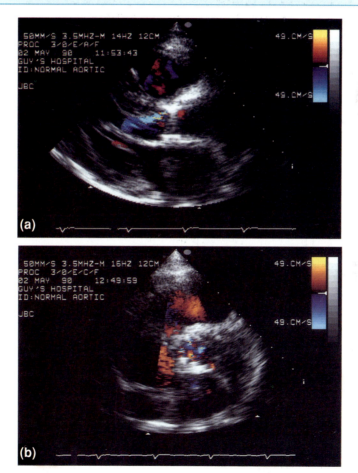

Figure 5.3: Normal pivotal washing jets in a bileaflet mechanical valve in the aortic position. In the parasternal long-axis view (a) the jet looks spuriously paraprosthetic because of its origin towards the edge of the sewing ring. The true situation is revealed in a modified short-axis view (b) where four jets can be seen, two from the upper and two from the lower pivotal point

REPORTING PROSTHETIC VALVES

1. **Valve position and type**
2. **Any signs of obstruction**
3. **Regurgitation, site and degree**
4. **Doppler forward flow values**
5. **Left ventricular dimensions and function**

COMMON MISTAKES

Missed mitral regurgitation

Shielding of ultrasound by the mechanical parts of the valve may cause failure to image the intra-atrial portion of a jet. Flow recruitment within the left ventricle is usually visible, but if there is doubt, transesophageal examination is necessary.

Overdiagnosing aortic obstruction

Surprisingly high transaortic pressure differences may be found in normally functioning valves, especially size 19 mm and 21 mm stented porcine or tilting disc valves (normal ranges on pages 74–78). For a mechanical valve, obstruction in the aortic position is much less common than in the mitral position. Provided that the patient is well, pathological obstruction should not be overdiagnosed.

Overdiagnosis of paraprosthetic aortic regurgitation

The pivotal washing jets of bileaflet mechanical prostheses have their origin close to the sewing ring and may be mistaken for paraprosthetic regurgitation. If in doubt, check the parasternal short-axis view. A normal jet will usually be accompanied by others and will be clearly within the orifice (Figure 5.3, page 41). Careful scanning at the level of the sewing ring will show the origin of a paraprosthetic jet outside the sewing ring.

REFERENCE

1. Chambers J, Fraser A, Lawford P, *et al*. Echocardiographic assessment of artificial heart valves: British Society of Echocardiography Position Paper. *Br Heart J* 1994; 71 (Suppl): 6–14

6

The right heart including pulmonary pressures

RIGHT VENTRICLE

1. Is the right ventricle enlarged?

Right ventricular dilatation is present if it is as large as, or larger than, the left in the apical 4-chamber view. Normal dimensions are given in Table A2.4, page 73.

Do not overdiagnose right ventricular enlargement using oblique parasternal cuts.

2. If large, is the right ventricle active or hypokinetic?

- An active dilated right ventricle suggests left-to-right shunt or tricuspid or pulmonary regurgitation.

- A dilated, hypokinetic right ventricle suggests a right ventricular myopathy, infarction or acute or end-stage chronic valve disease or pulmonary hypertension.

- If there is a regional abnormality of contraction, look at the inferior wall of the left ventricle for an infarct (Figure 6.1).

3. Is there right ventricular hypertrophy?

Hypertrophy is defined by a free wall thickness exceeding 4 mm. It suggests pulmonary hypertension, pulmonary stenosis, hypertrophic cardiomyopathy or amyloid.

4. Is there any left-sided valve disease?

Pulmonary hypertension as a result of severe mitral stenosis may result in right ventricular dilatation.

43

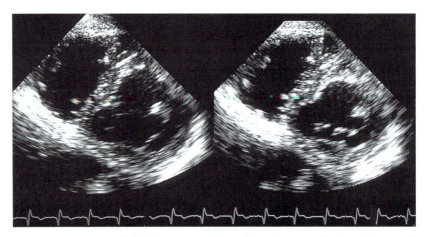

Figure 6.1: Myocardial infarction involving the right ventricle: the inferior wall of the left ventricle is thin and akinetic. The adjacent right ventricular wall is also infarcted and does not thicken between diastole (left) and systole (right)

5. **Is there evidence of a shunt above the right ventricle?**

If the right ventricle is dilated and active but no fossa ovalis atrial septal defect is visible, consider a sinus venosus atrial septal defect or partial anomalous pulmonary venous drainage.

6. **Check for tricuspid regurgitation and pulmonary regurgitation (*see* below)**

7. **What is the pulmonary artery pressure? (*see* page 49)**

8. **You should now be able to suggest the likely cause of right ventricular dilatation (Table 6.1)**

Table 6.1 Causes of right ventricular dilatation

Left-to-right shunt above the right ventricle
Pulmonary hypertension
   secondary to mitral valve disease
   secondary to chronic left-to-right shunts
   secondary to pulmonary emboli or lung disease
   primary
Tricuspid or pulmonary regurgitation
Right ventricular infarction
Right ventricular myopathy

TRICUSPID VALVE DISEASE

1. Is there tricuspid regurgitation?

Is it mild, moderate or severe?

Jet area on color mapping is smaller than for an equivalent degree of mitral regurgitation because driving pressures are lower for the right than the left heart in the absence of severe pulmonary hypertension.

In torrential tricuspid regurgitation, the map may be of low velocity and broad, but the continuous-wave Doppler signal may have a triangular shape resembling semilunar valve flow (Figure 6.2).

Other guides to severity are a dilated inferior vena cava, large right atrium and holosystolic flow reversal in the hepatic veins.

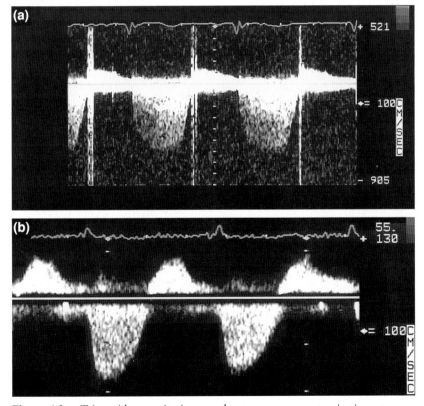

Figure 6.2: Tricuspid regurgitation: moderate or severe regurgitation causes a large intra-atrial jet on color mapping with a continuous-wave signal which retains its usual shape (a). In torrential regurgitation, the color map may show homogeneous reverse flow and the continuous-wave signal (b) will then resemble that obtained from the pulmonary or aortic valves

2. What is the etiology of the tricuspid regurgitation?

Rheumatic disease is easily missed since there is little leaflet thickening, in contrast to left-sided valves. Bowing of the valve as a result of commissural fusion may be obvious (Figure 6.3).

Carcinoid causes stubby, retracted leaflets and also affects the pulmonary valve.

Other causes of organic disease are given in Table 6.2.

Is there another cause for regurgitation, e.g. annular dilatation or a pacing electrode?

Table 6.2   Causes of tricuspid regurgitation

Valve disease
    rheumatic disease
    myxomatous degeneration
    endocarditis
    carcinoid
    congenital (e.g. Ebstein's anomaly)
    amyloid

Functional abnormalities
    pulmonary hypertension
    right ventricular dilatation
    artificial pacing

---

3. What is the estimated pulmonary artery pressure? (*see* page 49)

4. Is tricuspid stenosis present? (Figure 6.3)

This is suggested by a peak velocity > 1.5 m/s in the absence of severe tricuspid regurgitation. The pressure half-time is also prolonged in severe stenosis but may vary with respiration, particularly in more mild stenosis. Another clue is a small right ventricle (because of underfilling) and large right atrium (because of high back pressure).

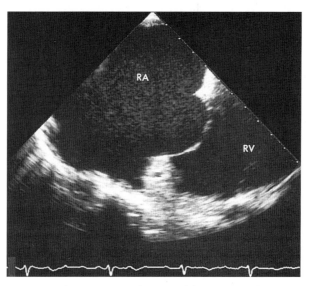

Figure 6.3: Tricuspid stenosis may be missed because, unlike the mitral valve, there is little thickening or calcification. Doming during diastole occurs as a result of commissural fusion (in this example on transesophageal examination). Stenosis is confirmed by an elevation in peak velocity (in the absence of significant regurgitation which will produce the same effect). RA, right atrium; RV, right ventricle

PULMONARY VALVE DISEASE

1. Is there pulmonary regurgitation?

Assess its severity using the width of the jet on color flow Doppler and the length of diastolic flow reversal in the pulmonary artery. Trivial or mild pulmonary regurgitation is normal.

2. What is the etiology?

Are the leaflets abnormal (Table 6.3) or is the regurgitation secondary to pulmonary hypertension?

3. Is there pulmonary stenosis?

Even in severe stenosis, valve thickening may be minimal. The most obvious initial clue is turbulent, high-velocity flow in the pulmonary artery during systole on color Doppler mapping.

Table 6.3   Etiology of pulmonary regurgitation

Congenital
Pulmonary hypertension
Carcinoid
Endocarditis
Following pulmonary valvotomy

What is the pressure difference across the valve? A difference of 50 mmHg is a frequently-applied threshold for severe pulmonary stenosis assuming normal right ventricular systolic function.

4. What is the pulmonary artery pressure? (*see* below)

This is relevant if there is dominant pulmonary regurgitation which may be caused by pulmonary hypertension.

Pulmonary stenosis tends to protect the pulmonary circulation against the effect of high flow from a left-to-right shunt.

A normal diastolic pressure associated with a moderately raised systolic pressure in the presence of a left-to-right shunt may occur as a result of high flow rather than established pulmonary hypertension.

ESTIMATING PULMONARY ARTERY PRESSURE

Systolic

1. Measure the maximum peak instantaneous velocity (v) of the tricuspid regurgitant signal. From this, estimate the gradient across the tricuspid valve using the short form of the modified Bernoulli equation ($4v^2$).

2. Estimate the right atrial pressure. The most reliable method is the semi-subjective technique of assessing contraction of the inferior vena cava during inspiration (Table 6.4). The inferior vena cava is imaged subcostally and its diameter is examined 1 cm before it joins the right atrium.

3. Pulmonary artery systolic pressure is the sum of (1.) and (2.), assuming that there is no pulmonary stenosis.

Table 6.4 Semi-subjective estimation of right atrial pressure from inferior vena cava

Diameter on expiration (cm)	Collapse on inspiration (%)	Pressure estimate (mmHg)
< 2	complete	0–5
< 2	> 50	5–10
> 2	25–50	10–15
> 2	< 25	15–20

Diastolic

1. Measure the end-diastolic velocity of the pulmonary regurgitant signal (Figure 6.4).
   From this, estimate the gradient across the pulmonary valve using the short form of the modified Bernoulli equation ($4v^2$).

2. Estimate the right atrial pressure (Table 6.4).

3. Pulmonary artery diastolic pressure is the sum of (1.) and (2.).

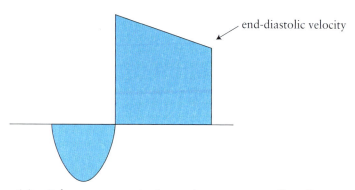

Figure 6.4: Pulmonary regurgitation: pulmonary artery diastolic pressure is estimated using the end-diastolic velocity of the pulmonary regurgitant continuous-wave signal (arrow). This is then entered into the modified Bernoulli equation ($4v^2$) and added to an estimate of right atrial pressure

RIGHT ATRIAL MASS

1. Is the mass normal?

A prominent eustachian valve may be mistaken for an abnormal mass. A chiari net or atrial septal aneurysm may also be misdiagnosed.

2. If abnormal, what is the size, shape and density of mass?

3. Is it sessile or mobile?

Sessile masses are likely to be malignant. Mobile masses may be thrombus or myxoma.

4. Where is it attached?

- Attachment to the atrial septum suggests a myxoma although, occasionally, thrombus may become ensnared in a patent foramen ovale.
- Both tumor from kidneys or uterus and thrombus enter via the inferior vena cava.
- A sessile mass attached to the free wall of the right atrium suggests a malignant tumor.

5. Is the inferior vena cava filled with mass?

Thrombus tends to maintain a normal inferior vena cava size. Tumor causes dilatation of the inferior vena cava.

6. Is there a pericardial effusion?

This suggests angiosarcoma.

REPORTING THE RIGHT HEART

1. **Right ventricular dimensions**
2. **Right ventricular regional and global systolic function**
3. **Appearance and function of valves**
4. **Pulmonary artery pressure**
5. **Any masses?**

7

Aorta

As much of the thoracic and abdominal aorta as can be imaged should be examined in patients:

- With a widened mediastinal shadow on the chest radiograph.
- With suspected aortic dissection.
- Who are predisposed to aortic dilatation (e.g. Marfan Syndrome, Ehlers–Danlos Type IV).
- Who have an abnormal root dimension on M-mode.

1. What is the diameter of the aorta?

Measure the diameter at the following levels (Figure 7.1). Normal ranges are given in Table 7.1[1-5]:

- Annulus (parasternal long axis).
- Sinus of Valsalva (parasternal long axis).
- Sinotubular junction (parasternal long axis; right intercostal).
- Arch (suprasternal).
- Descending (suprasternal, apical, modified parasternal long axis).
- Abdominal (subcostal).

Table 7.1 Normal ranges for aortic diameter (cm)

Level (Figure 7.1)		Absolute	Indexed to BSA
A	annulus	1.7–2.5	1.1–1.5
B	sinus of Valsalva	2.2–3.6	1.4–2.0
C	sinotubular junction	1.8–2.6	1.0–1.6
D	arch	1.4–2.9	0.8–1.9
E	descending	1.1–2.3	0.8–1.2
F	abdominal	1.0–2.2	0.6–1.3

BSA, body surface area

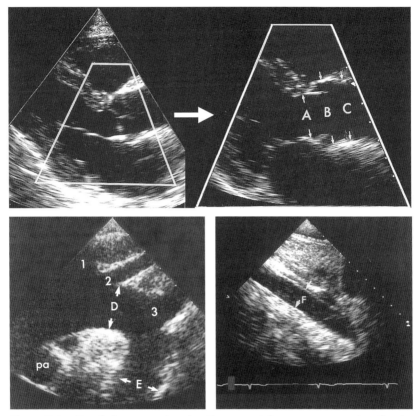

Figure 7.1: Levels for measuring the diameter of the aorta: conventionally, the annulus is measured from inner margin to inner margin (in the absence of significant reverberation artifact from a calcific aortic valve). Other dimensions are usually made from leading edge to leading edge. A, annulus; B, sinus of Valsalva; C, sinotubular junction; D, arch; E, descending thoracic; F, abdominal; 1, innominate artery; 2, left carotid artery; 3, left subclavian artery; pa, pulmonary artery

2. Is there a dissection flap?

An intraluminal flap is the hallmark of dissection, but transthoracic echocardiography has limited diagnostic power, especially in the descending thoracic aorta. If the transthoracic study is normal, consider transesophageal echocardiography.

3. Is there aortic regurgitation?

Dilatation of the ascending aorta is a cause of aortic regurgitation. Assessment of severity is described on pages 23–25.

4. If dissection is suspected, is there pericardial fluid?

This suggests rupture into the pericardial sac which is a common cause of death in acute dissection. It may suggest the diagnosis even if a flap cannot be imaged.

REPORTING THE AORTA

1. **Diameter at each level**
2. **Aortic regurgitation**
3. **Dissection flap**
4. **Pericardial effusion (if dissection is suspected)**

COMMON MISTAKES

Artifact mistaken for dissection flap

A flap causes an echo moving out of phase with the rest of the aorta (Figure 7.2a). Artifact is easily mistaken for a flap (Figure 7.2b), but causes linear echoes usually moving in phase with the aortic walls. The color Doppler flow patterns characteristic of dissection are also absent in association with artifact.

REFERENCES

1. Oh TK, Taliercio CP, Holmes DR, *et al*. Prediction of the severity of aortic stenosis by Doppler aortic valve area determination. *JACC* 1988; 11: 1227–34
2. Davidson WR, Pasquale MJ, Fanelli C. A Doppler echocardiographic examination of the normal aortic valve and left ventricular outflow tract. *Am J Cardiol* 1991; 67: 547–9
3. Schnittger I, Gordon EP, Fitzgerald PJ, *et al*. Standardized intracardiac measurements of two dimensional echocardiography. *JACC* 1983; 2: 934–8
4. Mintz GS, Kotler MN, Segal BL, *et al*. Two dimensional echocardiographic recognition of the descending thoracic aorta. *Am J Cardiol* 1979; 44: 232–8
5. Guy's Database. Guy's Hospital, London, UK. (unpublished data)

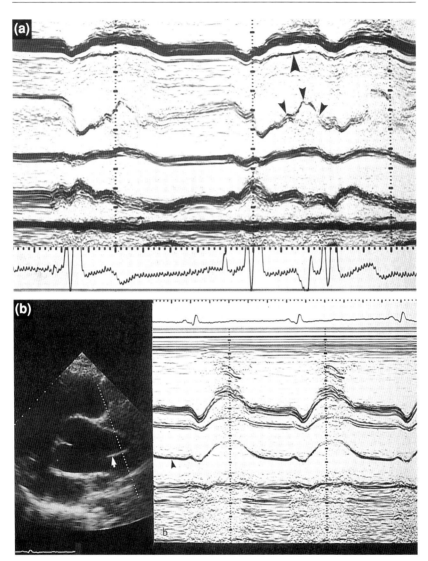

Figure 7.2: Echocardiography in suspected dissection: a true flap (a) has an irregular motion out of phase with the aorta and other structures. An artifact (b) tends to be linear and to move in phase with a structure in the normal heart, in this example with the right ventricular wall

8

Adult congenital disease

Atrial septal defect

- The diagnosis should be considered if the right ventricle is dilated.

- Describe the position (Figure 8.1). In adults, most are at the fossa ovalis.

- Calculate the shunt as the ratio of flow at the pulmonary artery to the aorta (Table 8.1).

- What is the pulmonary artery pressure (page 49).

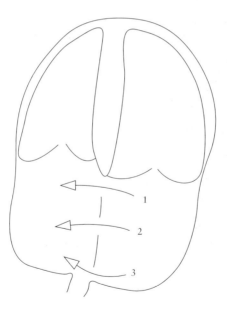

Figure 8.1: Position of atrial septal defects: in adults, the most common defect is the secundum (or fossa ovalis) defect (2), found in 75% of cases. Endocardial cushion defects (1) are found in around 10% and sinus venosus defects (3) in 10%. The latter arise when the roof of the superior vena cava (or occasionally the inferior vena cava) is incomplete

Table 8.1 Levels for shunt calculation

	Downstream	Upstream
Atrial septal defect	pulmonary artery	aorta
Ventricular septal defect	pulmonary artery	aorta
Persistent ductus	aorta	pulmonary valve

Ventricular septal defect

- Localize the site of the defect (Figure 8.2).

- Estimate the shunt (Table 8.1 and page 80). Left ventricular volume load suggests a large shunt.

- Estimate pulmonary artery pressures (page 49).

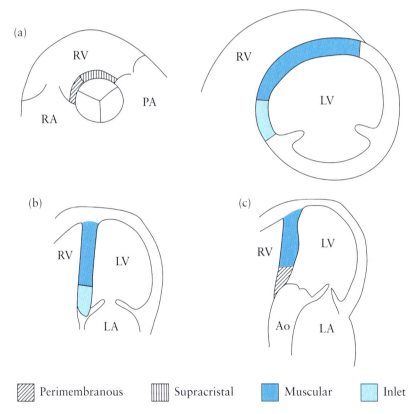

Perimembranous   Supracristal   Muscular   Inlet

Figure 8.2: Position of ventricular septal defects: (a) short axis; (b) apical 4-chamber; (c) apical 5-chamber. RV, right ventricle; RA, right atrium; PA, pulmonary artery; LV, left ventricle; LA, left atrium; Ao, aorta

Persistent ductus

- Look for reversed flow in the main pulmonary artery using the parasternal short axis as well as suprasternal view. If the shunt is small, flow may only be seen in diastole. Larger shunts are seen in systole as well as diastole and the size is approximately related to the width of abnormal flow on color mapping.

- Estimate the shunt (page 80) (Table 8.1). Left ventricular volume load suggests a large shunt.

- When pulmonary artery pressure is high, flow may diminish, cease or reverse during systole (Figure 8.3).

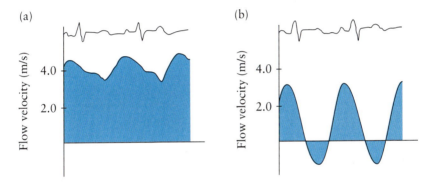

Figure 8.3: Flow patterns in persistent ductus: in a significant ductus (a), there is high velocity flow during both systole and diastole. With significant pulmonary hypertension, flow reduces or reverses during systole (b)

Coarctation

- The most important feature on continuous-wave recordings is forward flow during diastole.

- During systole, flow velocities are raised (Figure 8.4). However, if there is a severe coarctation with extensive collaterals, it may be difficult to obtain a clear systolic signal, but flow still continues throughout the cycle.

- Even after successful repair, systolic velocities are usually above normal but diastolic flow will not be seen.

Unknown diagnosis

Complex congenital disease is beyond the scope of this book. However, this is a guide to basic assessment:

- Make no assumptions about anatomy, but work systematically.

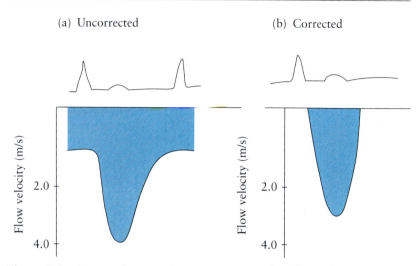

Figure 8.4: Coarctation: continuous-wave recording from the suprasternal position. There are elevated flow velocities in systole; forward flow continues throughout diastole (a). After successful correction, systolic velocities remain elevated but there is no abnormal diastolic forward flow (b)

- 'AV valve' refers to the tricuspid and mitral and 'semilunar valve' to the pulmonary and aortic. Thus, 'left AV valve' makes no assumptions that this is truly the mitral valve.

- 'Anatomical left ventricle' means the ventricle on the left of the heart; 'morphological left ventricle' means the ventricle attached to the mitral valve.

1. **Are atria attached to correct veins?**

2. **Are atria attached to correct ventricles?**

The morphological right ventricle is recognized because:

- Its valve is more apical than on the left.

- There is a gap between the AV valve and the semilunar valve.

- There are more trabeculations than in the morphological left ventricle.

3. **Are ventricles attached to correct great arteries?**

The pulmonary artery is recognized because it bifurcates early.

Transposition of the great vessels is present if both great vessels can be imaged in transverse section from a parasternal short-axis view.

4. Are there any shunts at atrial or ventricular level?

5. Are cardiac valves normal in appearance?

6. What is pulmonary artery pressure?

7. Is there aortic coarctation?

REPORTING CONGENITAL DISEASE

1. **Anatomy**
2. **Chamber size and function**
3. **Valve appearance and function**
4. **Shunts**
5. **Pulmonary artery pressure**

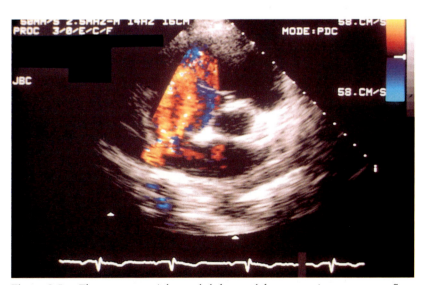

Figure 8.5: Flow across atrial septal defect and from superior vena cava: flow from the vena cava has an origin separate from flow across the atrial septum although both merge

COMMON MISTAKES

Superior vena cava flow mistaken for atrial septal defect

The entry of flow from these structures into the right atrium may be close (Figure 8.5). Take multiple views. If there is still doubt, the pulsed waveform may help. Flow across an atrial septal defect has a peak in late diastole and in systole. In the superior vena cava, the peaks are earlier (Figure 8.6).

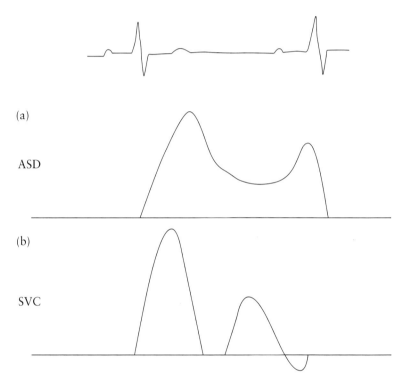

Figure 8.6: Pulsed Doppler waveform in atrial septal defect (ASD) and superior vena cava (SVC): in an atrial septal defect (a) there is biphasic flow with the higher velocity occurring in late systole in time with the atrial v wave and the second peak after atrial systole. In the superior vena cava (b), peak flow velocities occur earlier

9

Pericardial effusion

1. Pericardial or pleural? (Table 9.1 and Figure 9.1)

Table 9.1 Differential diagnosis of pericardial and pleural effusions

Pericardial	Pleural
Ends anterior to descending aorta	Ends posterior to descending aorta
Almost never overlaps left atrium	May overlap left atrium
Often between right ventricle and diaphragm on subcostal view	Never between right ventricle and diaphragm on subcostal view
Tamponade may be present	No signs of tamponade
Rarely > 4 cm in depth	May be > 4 cm in depth
Usually bobbing of heart	Heart fixed

2. Size and distribution

- Size is far less important than whether there are signs of tamponade (conventional measures of size are: small (1 cm), moderate (1–2 cm) and large (> 2 cm)).

- Is the effusion generalized/posterior/apical/anterior?

- Is there > 2 cm in the subcostal view (allowing safe pericardio-centesis)?

3. Is there evidence of tamponade?

Signs of tamponade are given in Table 9.2. Right atrial collapse occurs with small volumes of pericardial fluid and is too sensitive to suggest tamponade on its own.

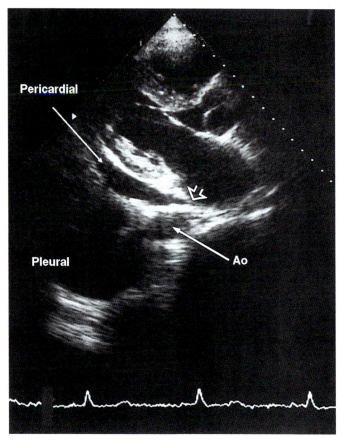

Figure 9.1: Pericardial versus pleural fluid: a pericardial effusion ends anterior to the descending thoracic aorta (Ao); a pleural effusion ends posterior to the aorta; a pleural effusion may extend over the left atrium, a pericardial effusion never does to any significant degree

Table 9.2 Echocardiographic evidence of tamponade

Dilated inferior vena cava (> 2 cm) with inspiratory collapse of < 50%
Fall in aortic or early diastolic mitral velocity during inspiration > 40%
Prolonged and widespread diastolic right ventricular collapse
Dominant systolic superior vena cava flow

Collapse of right atrium and right ventricular outflow tract are non-specific signs

4. General

- Is left ventricular function poor? (Pericardiocentesis may cause circulatory collapse.)

- If the effusion is small, but there is respiratory variability of left-sided velocities or the patient is significantly breathless, consider effusive–constrictive pericarditis (a mixture of effusion and pericardial constriction) (Table 1.11, page 12).

REPORTING PERICARDIAL EFFUSION

1. **Size and distribution**
2. **Evidence of tamponade**
3. **Is there enough fluid in the direction of proposed drainage?**
4. **Left ventricular function**

COMMON MISTAKES

Overdiagnosis of tamponade

Cardiac tamponade is failure of adequate cardiac output as a result of a pericardial effusion interfering with right and left ventricular filling. The signs of tamponade are given in Table 9.2. However, even a small pericardial effusion can produce abnormal signs in the absence of clinical tamponade, e.g. diastolic collapse of the right atrium or of the right ventricular outflow tract.

10

Other requests

Ejection systolic murmur

Assessments should include:

- Appearance and function of all valves including evidence of mitral prolapse.
- Pulmonary artery velocity.
- Ascending and descending aortic velocities for coarctation.
- Is there septal hypertrophy?
- Is there an atrial septal defect (if the right ventricle is large)?

Stroke

Transthoracic echocardiography has limited power in a patient with no clinical abnormality. Echocardiography can detect a direct source for emboli:

- Vegetation.
- Thrombus.
- Myxoma.

However, more usually echocardiography detects a condition with a known likelihood of thromboembolism, for example:

- Mitral stenosis.
- Dilated left ventricle.
- Dilated left atrium.

Suspected endocarditis

- Is there a vegetation?
- Is there a complication?

These are:

- Abscess.
- Fistula.
- Perforation.
- Aneurysm of a leaflet.
- Dehiscence of a replacement valve.

How much regurgitation is there?

Valve destruction is another sign of endocarditis. Obstruction is rare as a result of endocarditis.

Atrial fibrillation

Look for:

- Left ventricular dysfunction.
- Left ventricular hypertrophy.
- Mitral valve disease.
- Atrial size.
- Left atrial thrombus.
- Right ventricular dilatation.

Ventricular tachycardia

Look for:

- Left ventricular dysfunction.
- Left ventricular hypertrophy.
- Right ventricular dilatation.
- Floppy mitral valve.

Appendices

1. ORGANIZATION OF REPORT

Measurements

A report should have a section for objective M-mode or 2D dimensions and Doppler measurements displayed against appropriate normal ranges. Many pragmatic normal ranges are outdated, and modern data based on large populations include upper dimensions previously regarded as abnormal (*see* Appendix 2). Measurements of intracardiac dimensions can be useful in monitoring disease progression. These can be made using M-mode or 2D and must be interpreted in the light of the size and sex of the patient.

Text

This should include a description of observations made in a logical order which will vary for the operator and the study. The most important feature might be described first. Alternatively, each anatomical region might be discussed in turn.

Interpretation should not be a part of this section and even minor abnormalities are best described. These can be put into context in the conclusion. It is usually not advisable to describe each modality in turn or to describe findings at each window as is sometimes done. This is confusing, as small differences can emerge between different windows or repetitions may occur. It is better to integrate all windows and all modalities. Normal findings should also be stated and if a region could not be imaged this should also be admitted. This gives the reader the confidence that a systematic study has been undertaken rather than a study focused only on a region of interest.

Conclusion

This should summarize the whole study and be easily understood by a non-echocardiographer. It should identify any abnormality, its cause and any secondary effect. No interpretation not possible from the recorded study should be offered and no medical advice should be given.

2. NORMAL RANGES FOR CARDIAC DIMENSIONS (Figure A.1)

M-Mode:

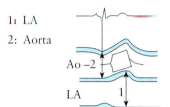

1: LA

2: Aorta

3: IVS in diastole
4: PW in diastole
5: diameter of LV in diastole
6: diameter of LV in systole

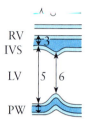

Figure A.1: Sites for making M-mode measurements: measurements are made from leading edge to leading edge. Diastolic measurements are timed with the onset of the QRS complex of the electrocardiogram. Left atrial (LA) diameter is taken as the maximum possible at the end of ventricular systole. Left ventricular (LV) systolic measurements are made at peak septal deflection when septal motion is normal or at peak posterior wall (PW) deflection in the presence of abnormal septal motion. Ao, aorta; IVS, interventricular septum; RV, right ventricle

Table A2.1 Normal intracardiac dimensions (cm) in men and women aged 18–72 years, 150–203 cm (59–80 ins) in height[1,2]

	Men	Women
LA	3.0–4.5, $n = 288$	2.7–4.0, $n = 524$
LVDD	4.3–5.9, $n = 394$	4.0–5.2, $n = 643$
LVSD	2.6–4.0, $n = 288$	2.3–3.5, $n = 524$
IVS (diastole)	0.6–1.3, $n = 106$	0.5–1.2, $n = 109$
PW (diastole)	0.6–1.2, $n = 106$	0.5–1.1, $n = 119$

LV, left ventricle; PW, posterior wall; LVDD, left ventricular diastolic dimension; LVSD, left ventricular systolic dimension; LA, left atrium; IVS, interventricular septum

Table A2.2 Upper 95% limit of intracardiac dimensions (cm) by height (m)[1,3]

	Height (m)									
	1.41–1.45	1.46–1.50	1.51–1.55	1.56–1.60	1.61–1.65	1.66–1.70	1.71–1.75	1.76–1.80	1.81–1.85	1.86–1.90
M-mode										
Male										
LVDD			5.3	5.4	5.5	5.5	5.6	5.7	5.8	5.9
LVSD			3.6	3.7	3.7	3.8	3.8	3.9	3.9	4.0
Female										
LVDD	4.9	4.9	5.0	5.1	5.1	5.2	5.3	5.3		
LVSD	3.1	3.2	3.3	3.3	3.4	3.4	3.5	3.5		
Two-dimensional										
Ann	2.0	2.0	2.1	2.1	2.2	2.2	2.3	2.3	2.4	2.4
LA	3.2	3.3	3.4	3.4	3.5	3.6	3.6	3.7	3.8	3.9

LVDD, left ventricular diastolic dimension; LVSD, left ventricular systolic dimension; Ann, aortic annulus; LA, left atrium

Table A2.3   Left ventricular cavity dimensions (cm) on 2D echocardiography by body surface area (m^2)[4]. (*See* Figure A.2 for site of measurement)

	Body surface area (m^2)		
	1.4–1.6	1.6–1.8	1.8–2.0
1 *Parasternal LA*			
Diastole	3.4–4.9	3.6–5.1	3.9–5.3
Systole	2.3–3.9	2.4–4.1	2.5–4.4
2 *Parasternal SA mitral level*			
Diastole	3.7–5.4	3.9–5.7	4.1–6.0
Systole	2.6–4.0	2.8–4.3	2.9–4.4
3 *Parasternal SA papillary*			
Diastole	3.5–5.5	3.8–5.8	4.1–6.1
Systole	2.3–3.9	2.4–4.0	2.6–4.1
4 *4-chamber mediolateral*			
Diastole	3.9–5.4	4.0–5.6	4.1–5.9
Systole	2.7–4.5	2.9–4.7	3.1–4.9
5 *4-chamber long-axis*			
Diastole	5.9–8.3	6.3–8.7	6.6–9.0
Systole	4.5–6.9	4.6–7.4	4.6–7.9

LA, long-axis; SA, short-axis

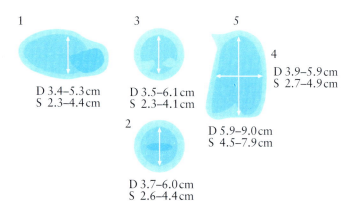

Figure A.2:   Sites for making 2D measurements. D, diastole; S, systole

Table A2.4   Right-sided dimensions (cm)*, upper 95% limit of normal[5]

Right ventricle systole	3.7
Right ventricle diastole	4.3
Right atrium	3.5

*Maximal transverse diameter in 4-chamber view

Table A2.5   Cardiac dimensions (cm) in athletic individuals (95% limits)[6]

	Male (n = 738)	Female (n = 209)
LA	3.1–4.3	2.8–4.0
LVDD	4.6–6.2	4.1–5.6
IVS (diastole)	0.8–1.3	0.7–1.0
PW (diastole)	0.8–1.1	0.6–1.1

LA, left atrium; LVDD, left ventricular disatolic dimension; IVS, interventricular septum; PW, posterior wall

3. NORMAL RANGES FOR PEAK BLOOD FLOW IN GREAT VESSELS[7]

Table A3.1   Great vessel peak blood flow (m/s)

Ascending aorta	0.7–1.4
Descending aorta	0.7–1.4
Abdominal	0.5–1.7
Pulmonary artery	0.5–1.2

4. NORMAL RANGES FOR REPLACEMENT HEART VALVES

These data are intended to be a guide to what is normal for different valve types in the aortic and mitral positions. However, many of the values are based on very small numbers of patients and interpretation must be made within the clinical context (symptoms, left ventricular function, regurgitation, previous findings).

The figures quoted are means with the standard deviation in brackets[8].

Table A4.1 Aortic position – biological

	Vmax (m/s)	MnΔP (mmHg)	EOA (cm^2)
Homograft			
22 mm	1.7 (0.3)	5.8 (3.2)	2.0 (0.6)
26 mm	1.4 (0.6)	6.8 (2.9)	2.4 (0.7)
Porcine			
Carpentier–Edwards			
21 mm	2.8 (0.5)		1.2 (0.2)
23 mm	2.8 (0.7)		1.1 (0.2)
25 mm	2.6 (0.6)		1.2 (0.3)
27 mm	2.5 (0.5)		1.3 (0.3)
29 mm	2.4 (0.4)		1.4 (0.1)
Intact			
21 mm	1.0 (0.1)	19.3 (7.4)	1.5 (0.3)
23 mm	1.3 (0.1)	18.8 (6.1)	1.6 (0.3)
25 mm	1.4 (0.2)	18.8 (8.0)	1.9 (0.3)
27 mm		15.0 (3.7)	
Hancock			
23 mm		12.0 (2.0)	
25 mm	2.4 (0.4)	11.0 (2.0)	
27 mm	2.4 (0.4)	10.0 (3.0)	
Bovine pericardial			
Labcor–Santiago			
19 mm		10.1 (3.1)	1.3 (0.1)
21 mm		8.2 (4.5)	1.3 (0.1)
23 mm		7.8 (2.9)	1.8 (0.2)
25 mm		6.8 (2.0)	2.1 (0.3)

Vmax, peak velocity; MnΔP, mean pressure difference; EOA, effective orifice area

Table A4.2   Aortic position – single tilting disk

	Vmax (m/s)	MnΔP (mmHg)	EOA (cm^2)
Bjork–Shiley			
21 mm	3.0 (0.9)		1.1 (0.3)
23 mm	2.4 (0.5)	14 (7.0)	1.3 (0.3)
25 mm	2.1 (0.5)	13.0 (5.0)	1.4 (0.4)
27 mm	2.0 (0.3)	10.0 (2.0)	1.6 (0.3)
Medtronic Hall			
21 mm		13.0 (4.0)	1.4 (0.1)
23 mm	2.3 (0.9)		
25 mm	2.1 (0.3)		
Omnicarbon			
21 mm	3.0 (0.3)	20.0 (5.0)	
23 mm	2.7 (0.3)	18.0 (5.0)	
25 mm	2.5 (0.3)	15.0 (4.0)	
27 mm	2.1 (0.2)	12.0 (2.0)	

Table A4.3   Aortic position – bileaflet

	Vmax (m/s)	MnΔP (mmHg)	EOA (cm^2)
St Jude			
19 mm	3.0 (0.6)	19.4 (7.2)	1.0 (0.3)
21 mm	2.6 (0.3)	14.8 (4.3)	1.3 (0.2)
23 mm	2.5 (0.5)	13.5 (5.9)	1.3 (0.3)
25 mm	2.4 (0.5)	12.2 (5.9)	1.8 (0.4)
27 mm	2.2 (0.5)	11.0 (5.0)	2.4 (0.6)
29 mm	2.0 (0.1)	7.0 (1.0)	2.7 (0.3)
Carbomedics			
19 mm	3.2 (0.4)	19.3 (8.5)	0.9 (0.3)
21 mm	2.5 (0.5)	13.7 (5.5)	1.3 (0.4)
23 mm	2.4 (0.4)	11.0 (4.6)	1.6 (0.4)
25 mm	2.3 (0.3)	9.1 (3.5)	1.8 (0.4)
27 mm	2.1 (0.4)	7.9 (3.4)	2.2 (0.6)
29 mm	1.8 (0.4)	5.6 (3.0)	3.2 (1.6)

Table A4.4   Aortic position – ball and cage

	Vmax (m/s)	MnΔP (mmHg)	EOA (cm²)
Caged ball			
Starr–Edwards			
23 mm	3.4 (0.6)		1.1 (0.2)
24 mm	3.6 (0.5)		1.1 (0.3)
26 mm	3.0 (0.2)		

Table A4.5   Mitral position – Porcine

	Vmax (m/s)	MnΔP (mmHg)	PHT (ms)
Carpentier–Edwards			
27 mm		6.0 (2.0)	95 (12)
29 mm	1.5 (0.3)	4.7 (2.0)	110 (30)
31 mm	1.5 (0.3)	4.5 (2.0)	102 (34)
33 mm	1.4 (0.2)	5.4 (4.0)	94 (26)
Intact			
25 mm		7.8 (2.4)	
27 mm		5.4 (1.5)	
Hancock			
29 mm		2.0 (0.7)	
31 mm		4.9 (1.7)	
33 mm		5.0 (2.0)	

PHT, pressure half time

Table A4.6   Mitral position – bovine pericardial

	Vmax (m/s)	MnΔP (mmHg)	PHT (ms)
Labcor–Santiago			
27 mm		2.8 (1.5)	85 (18)
29 mm		3.0 (1.3)	80 (34)

Table A4.7   Mitral position – single tilting disc

	Vmax (m/s)	MnΔP (mmHg)	PHT (ms)
Bjork–Shiley			
25 mm	1.6 (0.3)		
27 mm	1.5 (0.2)	2.7 (0.8)	94 (31)
29 mm	1.4 (0.4)	2.0 (0.1)	85 (22)
31 mm	1.5 (0.3)	3.4 (2.2)	81 (20)
33 mm	1.3 (0.6)		75 (25)
Medtronic–Hall			
29 mm	1.6 (0.1)		69 (15)
31 mm	1.5 (0.1)		77 (17)
Omnicarbon			
25 mm		6.0 (2.0)	
27 mm		6.0 (2.0)	
29 mm		5.0 (2.0)	
31 mm		6.0 (2.0)	

Table A4.8   Mitral position – bileaflet

	Vmax (m/s)	MnΔP (mmHg)	PHT (ms)
St Jude			
27 mm	1.6 (0.3)	5.0 (2.0)	
29 mm	1.6 (0.3)	4.5 (2.4)	81 (9)
31 mm	1.7 (0.4)	5.2 (3.0)	84 (12)
Carbomedics			
25 mm	1.6 (0.2)	4.3 (0.7)	92 (20)
27 mm	1.6 (0.3)	3.7 (1.5)	91 (24)
29 mm	1.8 (0.3)	3.7 (1.3)	79 (11)
31 mm	1.6 (0.4)	3.3 (1.1)	92 (20)
33 mm	1.4 (0.3)	3.4 (1.5)	79 (18)
Duromedics			
27 mm	1.9 (0.3)		105 (14)
29 mm	1.8 (0.2)		89 (18)
31 mm	1.7 (0.3)		99 (18)

Table A4.9   Mitral position – caged ball

	Vmax (m/s)	MnΔP (mmHg)	PHT (ms)
Starr–Edwards			
28 mm	1.8 (0.2)		130 (25)
30 mm	1.8 (0.2)		100 (40)
32 mm	1.9 (0.4)		125 (60)

5. SUMMARY OF FORMULAE

5.1 Bernoulli

This equates potential and kinetic energy up- and down-stream from a stenosis. The modified formula is used in two forms:

Short modified Bernoulli equation $\quad \Delta P = 4v_2^2$

Long modified Bernoulli equation $\quad \Delta P = 4(v_2^2 - v_1^2)$

where ΔP is transvalvar pressure difference (in mmHg), v_1 is subvalvar velocity (in m/s) and v_2 is transvalvar velocity in m/s.

The short form can be used when subvalvar is much less than trans-valvar velocity, e.g. mitral stenosis, moderate or severe aortic stenosis ($v_2 > 3.0$ m/s), but *not* mild aortic stenosis or normally functioning replacement valves.

5.2 Continuity equation

This is used in two forms:

Classical continuity equation $\quad \text{EOA} = \text{CSA} \times \text{vti}_1/\text{vti}_2$

Modified continuity equation $\quad \text{EOA} = \text{CSA} \times v_1/v_2$

where EOA is effective orifice area (in cm^2), CSA is cross-sectional area of the left ventricular outflow tract (in cm^2) and vti$_1$ and vti$_2$ are subaor-tic and transaortic systolic velocity time integral (in cm).

The modified form is a reasonable approximation in significant aortic stenosis, but not in mild stenosis or normally functioning replacement valves.

5.3 Pressure half-time

The pressure half-time orifice area formula is:

$$\text{MOA} = 220/T_{1/2}$$

where MOA is effective mitral orifice area (in cm^2) and $T_{1/2}$ is pressure half-time (in ms). This formula should only be used in moderate or severe stenosis. It has not been validated in normally functioning replace-ment valves.

5.4 Stroke volume

$$\text{SV} = \text{CSA} \times \text{vti}_1$$

where CSA is cross-sectional area of the left ventricular outflow tract (in cm^2) vti_1 is subaortic velocity time integral (in cm), and sv is stroke volume (in ml).

5.5 Shunt calculation

The stroke volume is calculated for the aortic valve as above and then for the right side at the level of either the pulmonary annulus or the main pulmonary artery. The shunt is then the ratio of pulmonary stroke volume to aortic stroke volume. (*See also* Table 8.1, page 58).

5.6 Flow

$$Flow \ (in \ ml/s) = CSA \times vti_1 \times 1000/SET$$

where CSA is cross-sectional area of the left ventricular outflow tract (in cm^2), vti_1 is subaortic velocity time integral (in cm) and SET is systolic ejection time (from opening to closing artifact of the aortic signal) (in ms).

5.7 Left ventricular (LV) mass

$$LV \ mass = 1.04 \times [(LVID + IVS + LVPW)^3 - LVID^3] - 13.6$$

where ID is internal diameter, IVS is interventricular septum and PW is posterior wall.

This is the Devereux formula which is widely applied, although it is not as accurate as 2D methods. It also uses the Penn convention of measurement taking the septal and posterior wall thicknesses from inner to inner edge. Using the American Society of Echocardiography (ASE) convention (i.e. leading edge to leading edge), the formula is:

$$LV \ mass = 0.83 \times [(LVID + IVS + LVPW)^3 - LVID^3] - 0.6.$$

When corrected for body surface area (*see* subsection 5.9), the upper limit for normal is $134 \ g/m^2$ for men and $110 \ g/m^2$ for women.

5.8 Two-dimensional determination of LV mass

There are two anatomically validated methods, the *area/length* and the *truncated ellipsoid* methods (Figure A.3). Both require the determination of the myocardial cross-sectional area at the level of the papillary muscle tips in the short-axis view. The epicardial and endocardial borders are traced to measure cross-sectional areas (A_1 and A_2, respectively). Assuming a circular cross-section, mean wall thickness can be calculated from mean outer and inner radius.

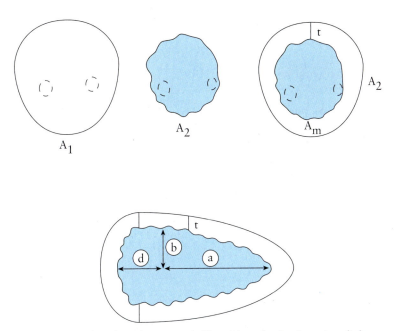

Figure A.3: Area/length and truncated ellipsoid methods. A_1, epicardial cross-sectional area; A_2, endocardial cross-sectional area; A_m, myocardial cross-sectional area; t, mean wall thickness; a, semi-major axis; b, short-axis; d, truncated semi-major axis radius

Both methods then use an apical 4-chamber and 2-chamber view to measure the major long axis. The area/length method uses the entire major axis whereas the truncated ellipsoid method divides the major axis into two parts at the level of the widest minor axis. These two segments are called the semi-major axis (a) and truncated semi-major axis (d).

The truncated ellipsoid and area/length formulae are contained within the sofware packages of most machines.

Body surface area

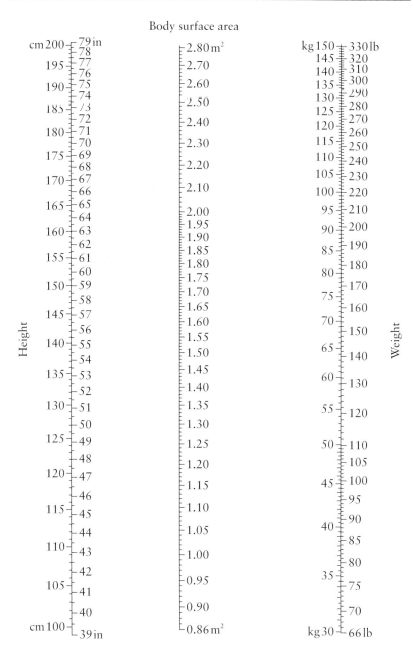

Figure A.4: Body surface area nomogram. Put a straight edge against the patient's height and weight and read off the body surface on the middle column. This is then divided into anatomic and physiologic parameters (e.g. LV mass, cardiac output) to correct for body habitus

6. EXAMPLES OF CONDITIONS REQUIRING URGENT CLINICAL ADVICE

Table A6.1

Postmyocardial infarction
    ventricular septal rupture
    severe mitral regurgitation
    pseudoaneurysm
Aortic dissection
Large pericardial effusion
Critical aortic stenosis
Myxoma or ball thrombus
Left ventricular thrombus or vegetation if there is evidence of peripheral embolization

REFERENCES

1. Lauer MS, Larson MG, Levy D. Gender specific reference M-mode values in adults: population-derived values with consideration of the impact of height. *JACC* 1995; 26: 1039–46
2. Devereux RB, Lutas EM, Casale PN, *et al*. Standardization of M-mode echocardiographic left ventricular anatomic measurements. *JACC* 1984; 4: 1222–30
3. Nidorf SM, Picard MH, Triulzi MO, *et al*. New perpectives in the assessment of cardiac chamber dimensions during development and adulthood. *JACC* 1992; 19: 983–8
4. Pearlman JD, Triulzi MO, King ME, *et al*. Limits of normal left ventricular dimensions in growth and development: analysis of dimensions and variance in the two dimensional echocardiograms of 268 normal healthy subjects. *JACC* 1988; 12: 1432–41
5. Triulzi MO, Gillam LD, Gentile F, *et al*. Normal adult cross-sectional echocardiographic values: linear dimensions and chamber areas. *Echocardiography* 1984; 1: 403–26
6. Pelliccia A, Maron BJ, Spataro A, *et al*. The upper limit of physiologic cardiac hypertrophy in highly trained elite athletes. *New Engl J Med* 1991; 324: 295–301
7. Wilson N, Goldberg SJ, Dickinson DF, *et al*. Normal intracardiac and great artery blood velocity measurements by pulsed Doppler echocardiography. *Br Heart J* 1985; 53: 451–8
8. Wang Z, Grainger N, Chambers J. Doppler echocardiography in normally-functioning replacement heart valves: a literature review. *J Heart Valve Dis* 1995; 4: 591–614

7. FURTHER READING

Basic introductory texts

- Halliwell M. Physics and principles. In Wilde P, ed. *Cardiac Ultrasound* Churchill Livingstone, 1993: 9–26

- Thirsk G. Equipment. In Wilde P, ed. *Cardiac Ultrasound*. Churchill Livingstone, 1993:27–40

- Fish P. *Physics and Instrumentation in Medical Ultrasound*. New York: John Wiley, 1990

- Labovitz AJ, Williams GA. *Doppler Echocardiography. The Quantitative Approach*. Lea and Febiger, 1992

- Jawad IA. *A Practical Guide to Echocardiography and Cardiac Doppler Ultrasound*, 2nd edn. Little, Brown and Co. 1996

- Monaghan MJ. *Practical Echocardiography and Doppler*. New York: John Wiley, 1990

- Chambers J. *Clinical Echocardiography*. BMJ Publications, 1995

Middle-range books

- Otto CM. *The Practice of Clinical Echocardiography*. Philadelphia: WB Saunders, 1997

- Kerut KK, McIlwain EF, Plotnick GD. *Handbook of Echo-Doppler Interpretation*. Futura Publishing Co, 1996

- Oh JK, Seward JB, Tajik AJ. *The Echocardiography Manual*. Little, Brown and Co, 1994

Advanced textbooks for reference

- Weyman AE. *Principles and Practice of Echocardiography*. 2nd edn. Lea and Febiger, 1994

- Feigenbaum H. *Echocardiography*, 5th edn. Lea and Febiger, 1994

Pediatric echocardiography

- Snider AR, Ritter SB, Sewer GA. *Echocardiography in Pediatric Heart Disease*. Mosby Year Book, 1997

General cardiology

- Lilly LS, ed. *Pathophysiology of Heart Disease*. Lea and Febiger, 1993
- Julian DG, Cowan JC. *Cardiology*, 6th edn. Eastbourne, UK: Ballière Tindall, 1992
- Braunwald E. *Heart Disease. A Textbook of Cardiovascular Medicine*, 5th edn. Philadelphia: WB Saunders, 1997
- Schlant RC, Alexander RW. *Hurst's the Heart*, 8th edn. New York: McGraw Hill, 1994

Index